世界髮型大全

HAIRSTYLES OF THE WORLD

LA COIFFURE AUTOUR DU MONDE · FRISUREN DER WELT
PEINADOS DEL MUNDO · ACCONCIATURE DEL MONDO
ESTILOS DE PENTEADO DO MUNDO

世界のヘアスタイル

D1532555

THE PEPIN PRESS

AMSTERDAM AND SINGAPORE

The Pepin Press publishes an extensive range of art books,
visual reference books, and practical design books.

Visit our websites for more information:
www.pepinpress.com
www.agilerabbit.com
www.webdesignindex.org

The Pepin Press BV
P.O. Box 10349
1001 EH Amsterdam, The Netherlands

Tel +31 20 4202021
Fax +31 20 4201152
mail@pepinpress.com

Concept and cover design by Pepin van Roojen
Research and layout by Dorine van den Beukel and Pepin van Roojen
Illustrations from The Pepin Press archive,
with additional illustrations by Joost Hölscher

ISBN 90 5496 082 5

10 9 8 7 6 5 4 3 2
2010 09 08 07 06 05 04 03

Printed in Singapore

Contents

ANTIQUITY

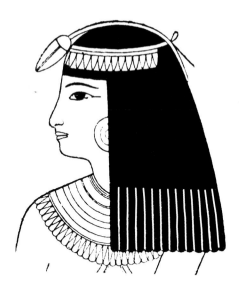

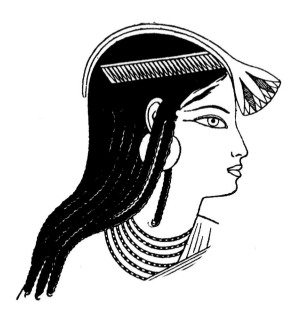

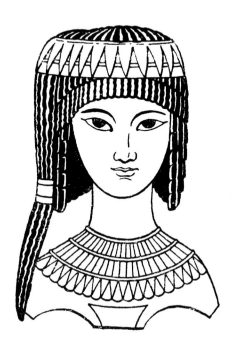

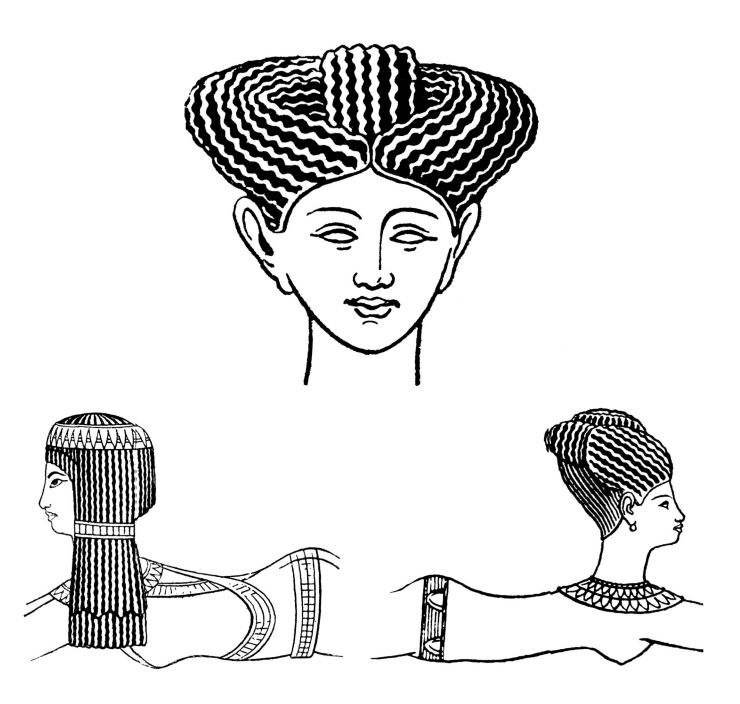

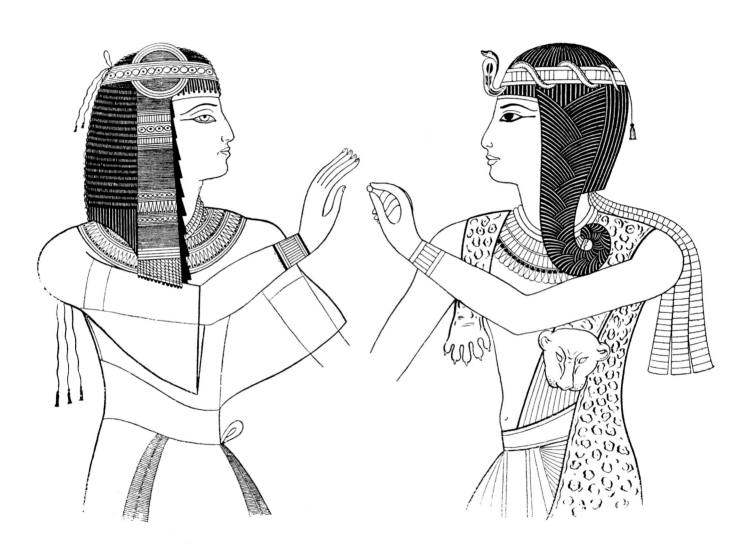

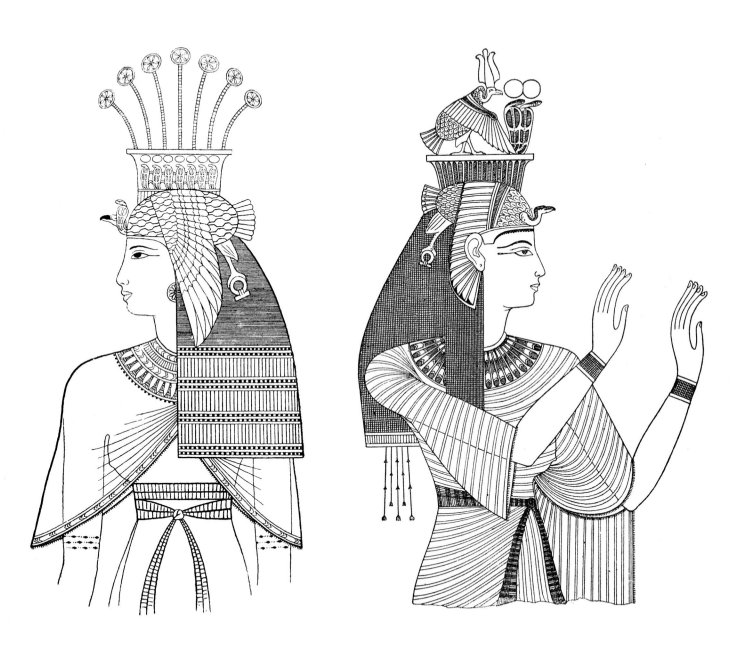

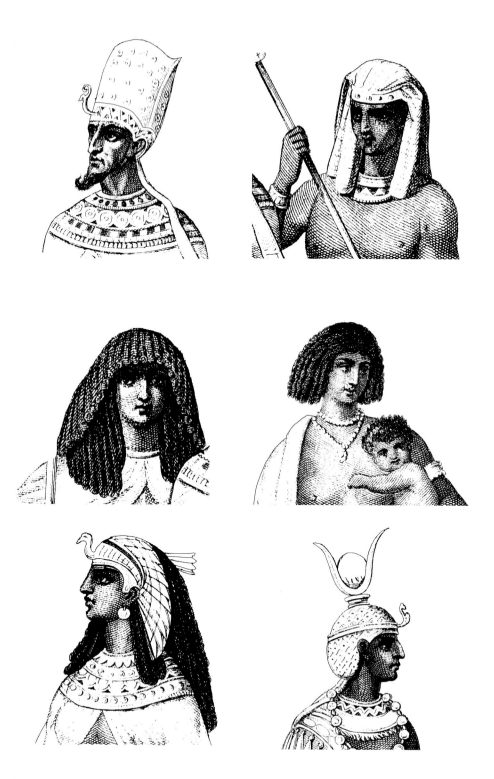

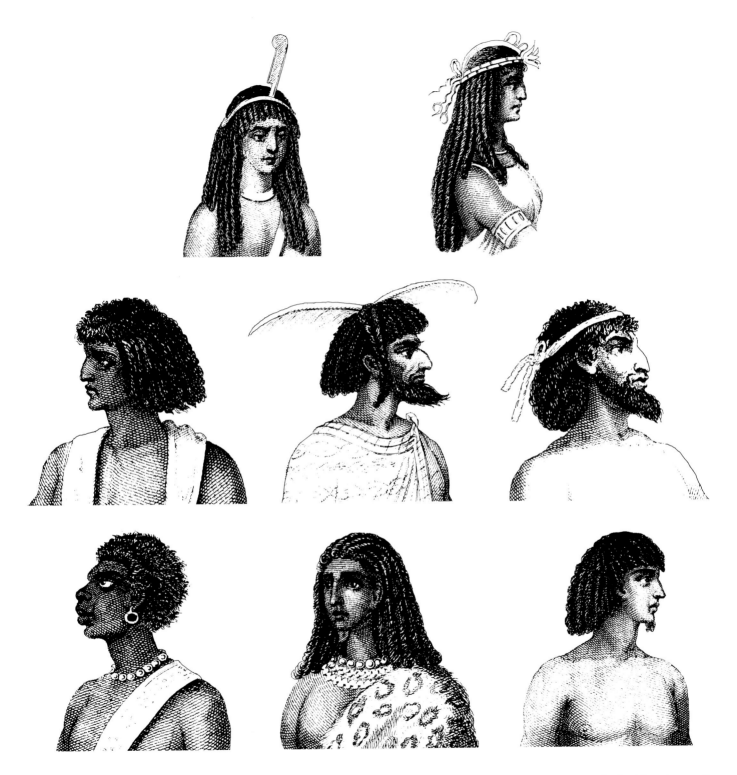

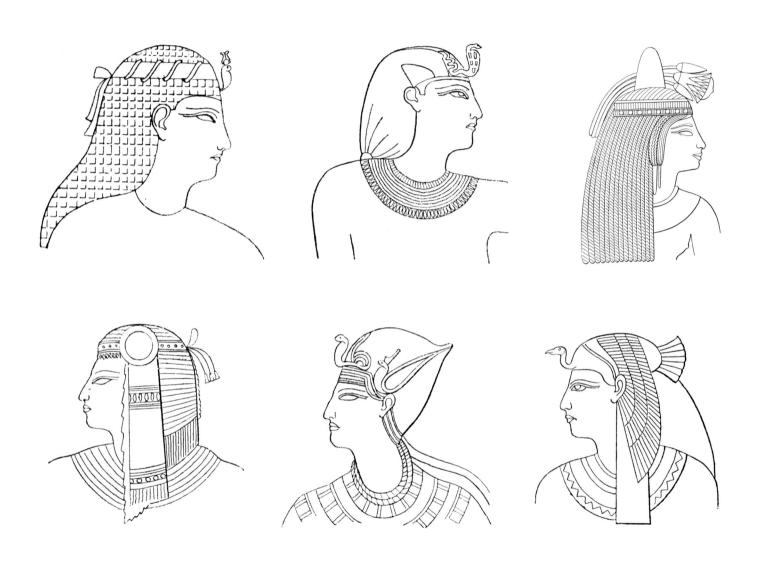

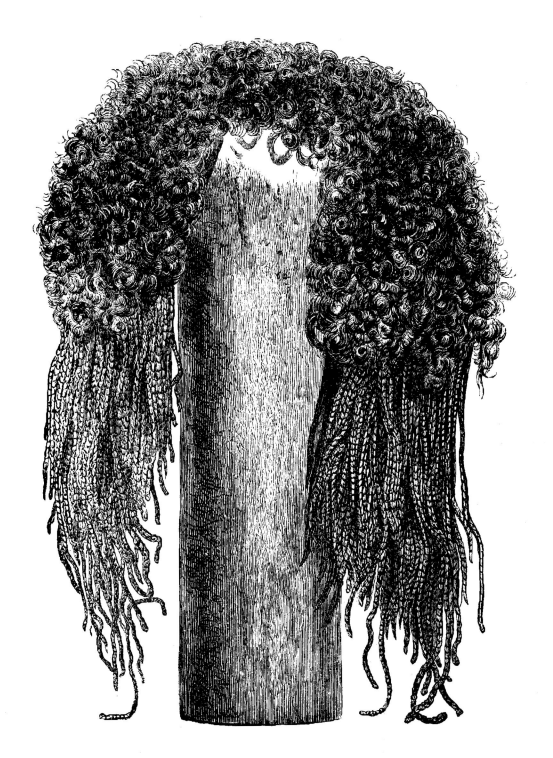

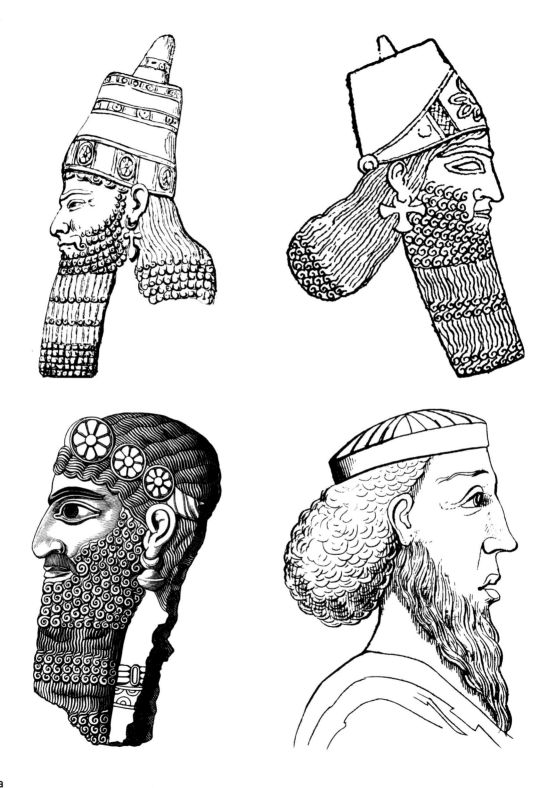

Assyria

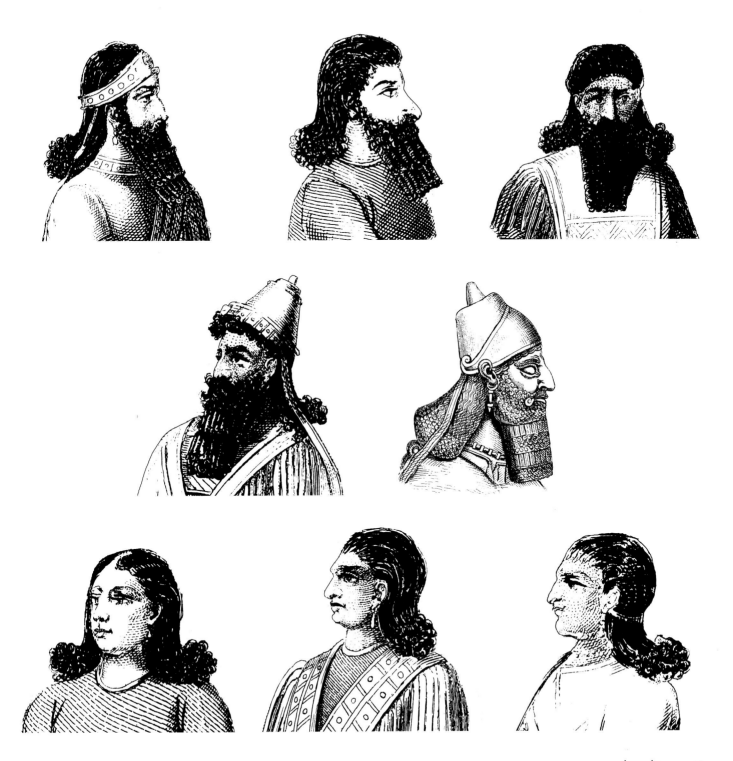

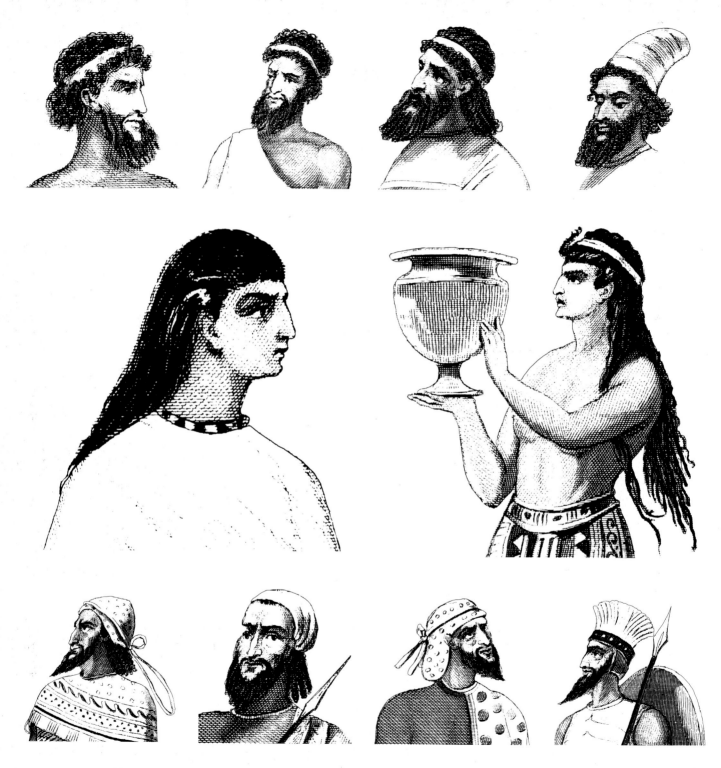

EUROPE

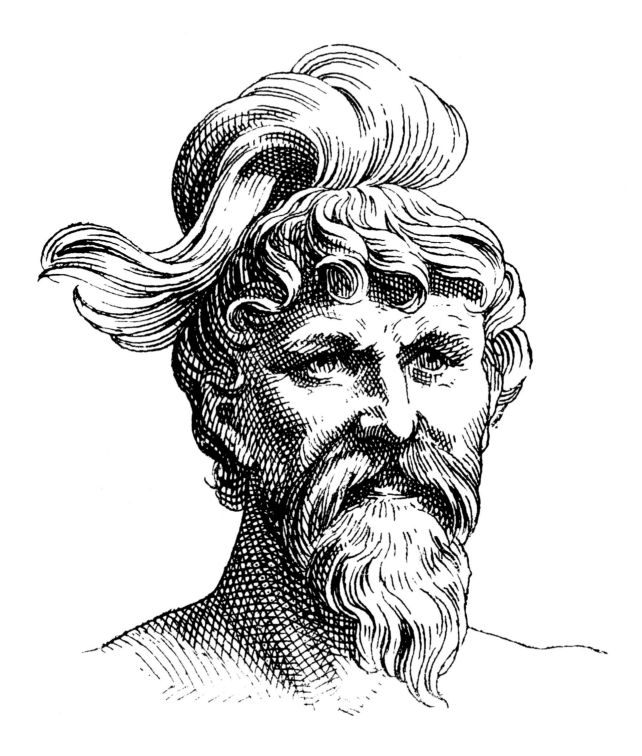

34   Germany, c. 300 AD

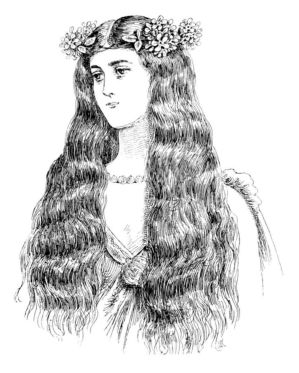

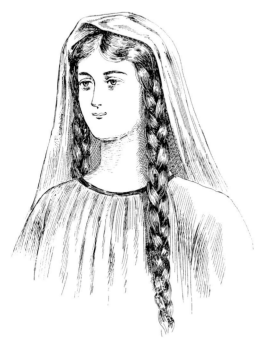

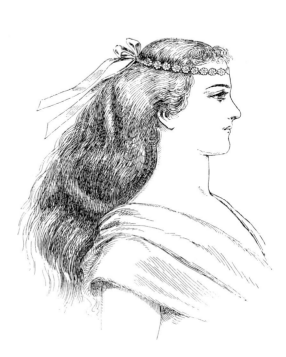

Scandinavia, c. 300 AD 35

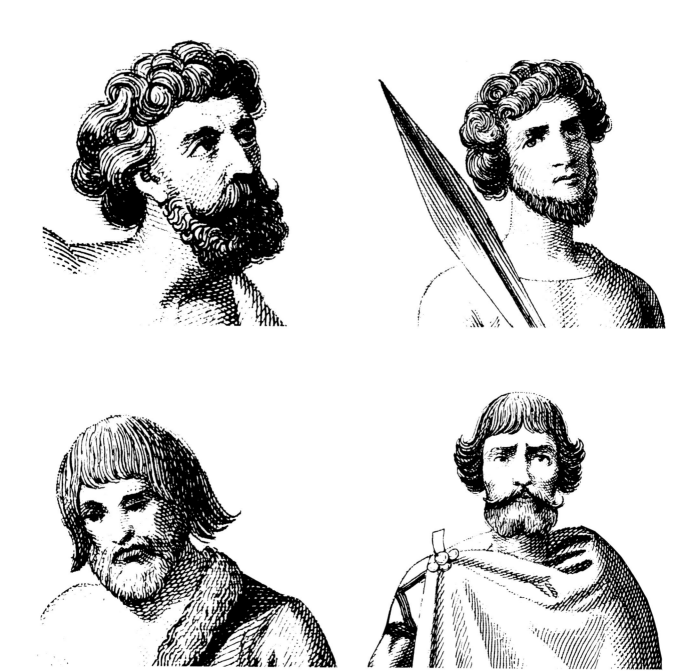

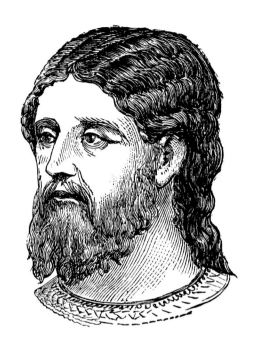

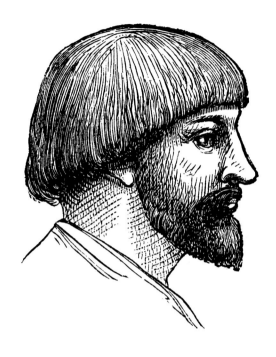

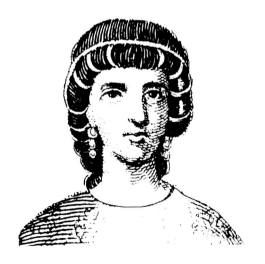

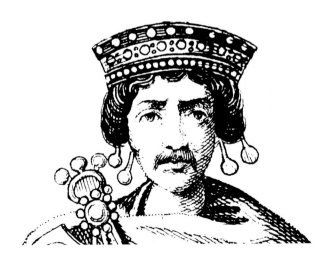

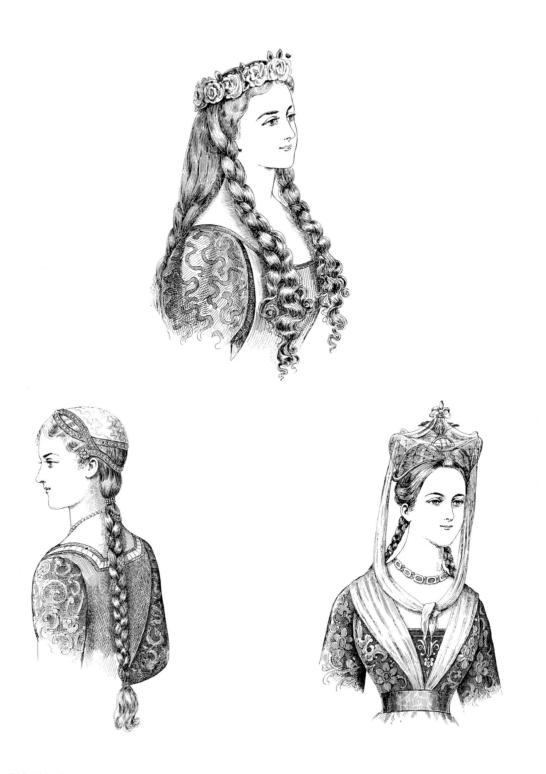

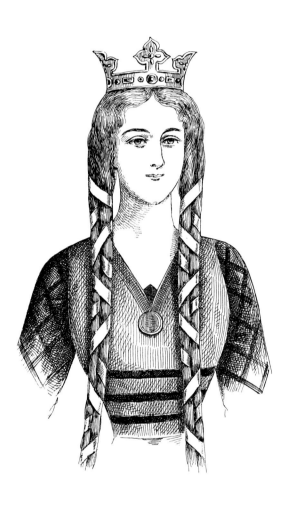 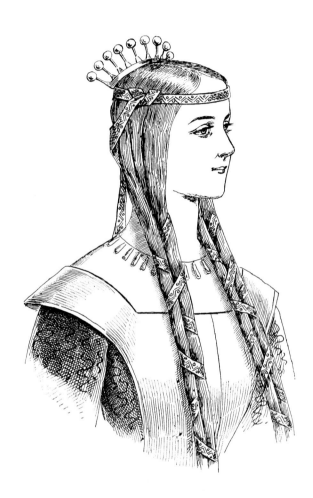

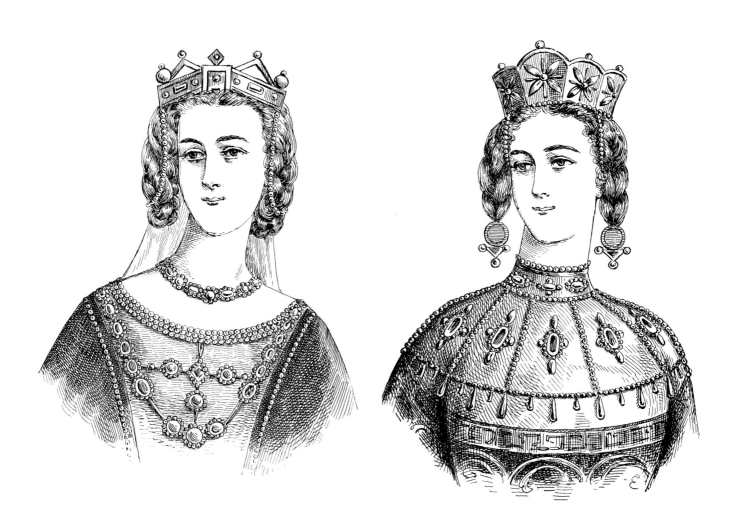

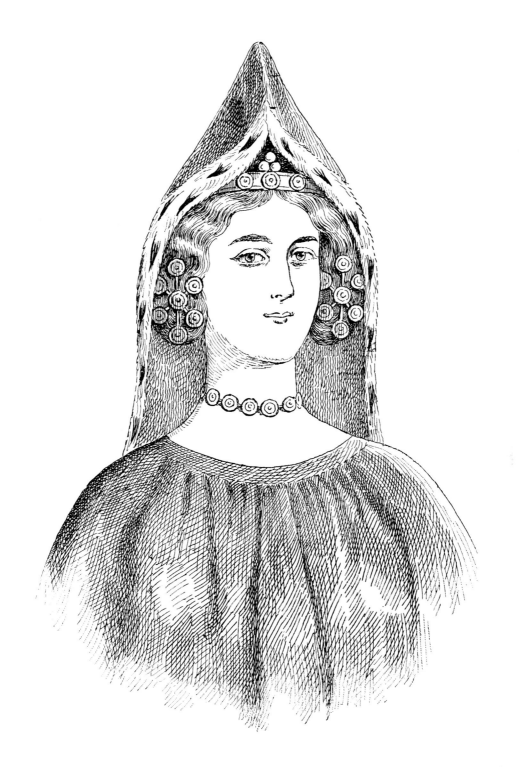

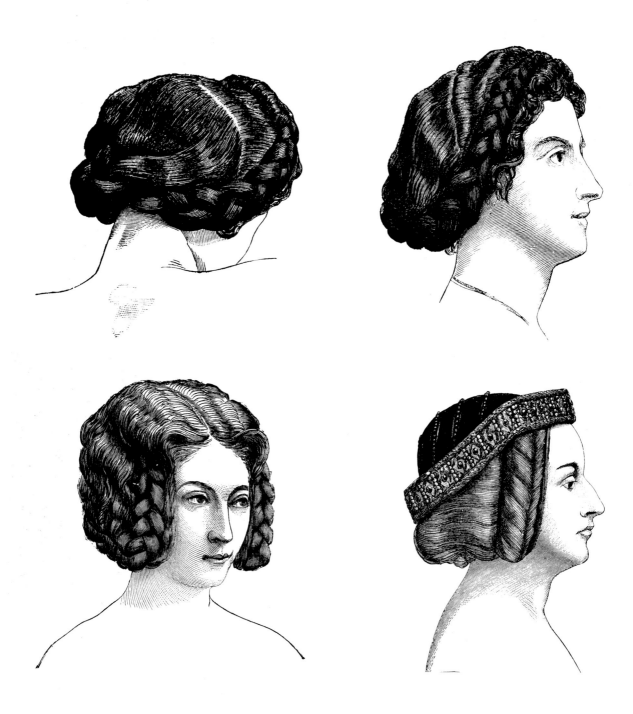

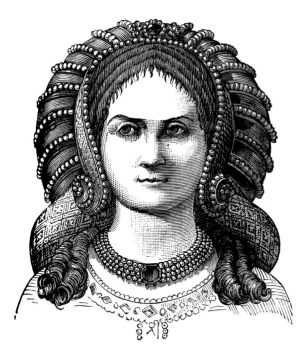

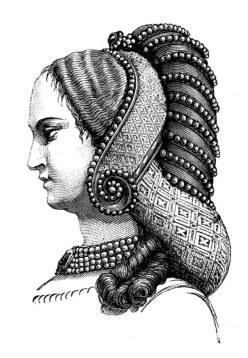

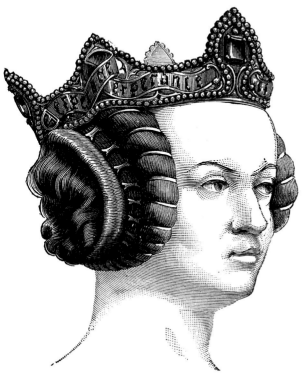

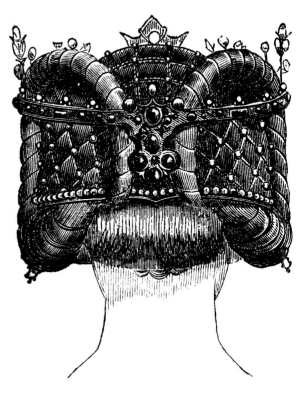

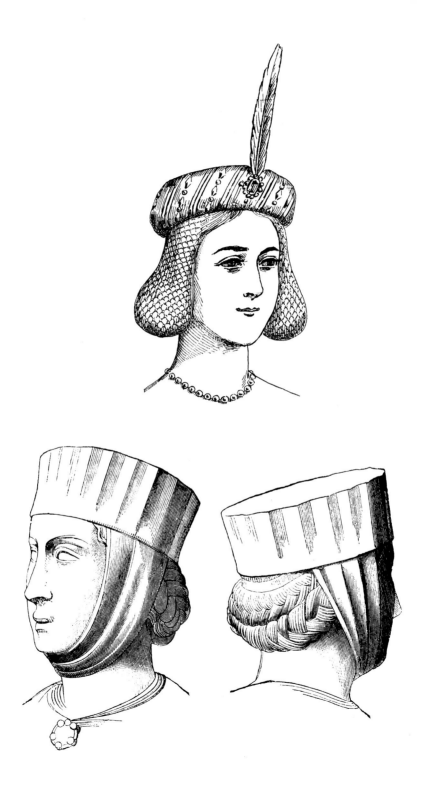

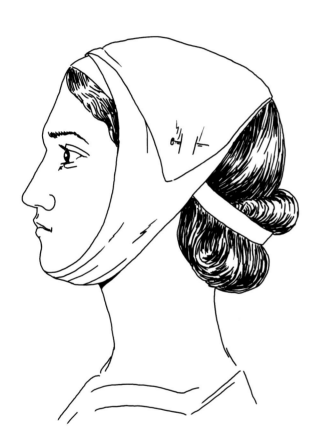
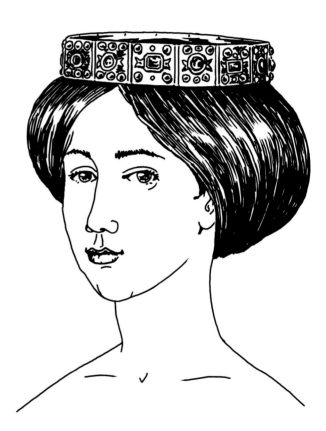

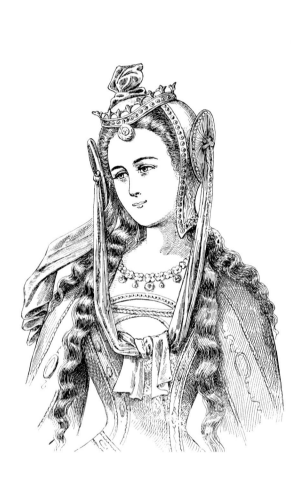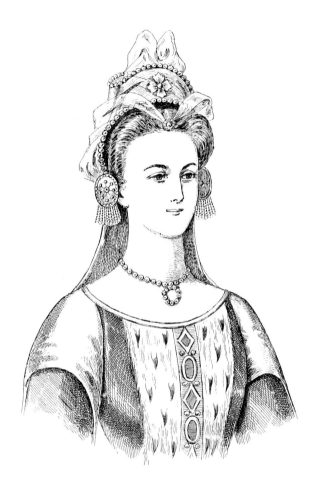

Europe. c. 1450

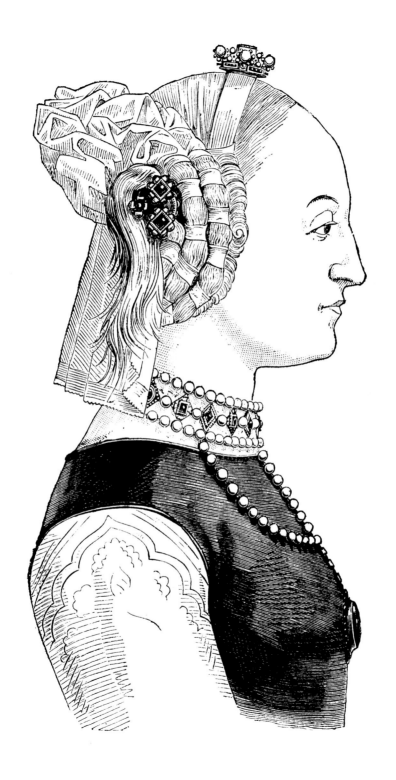

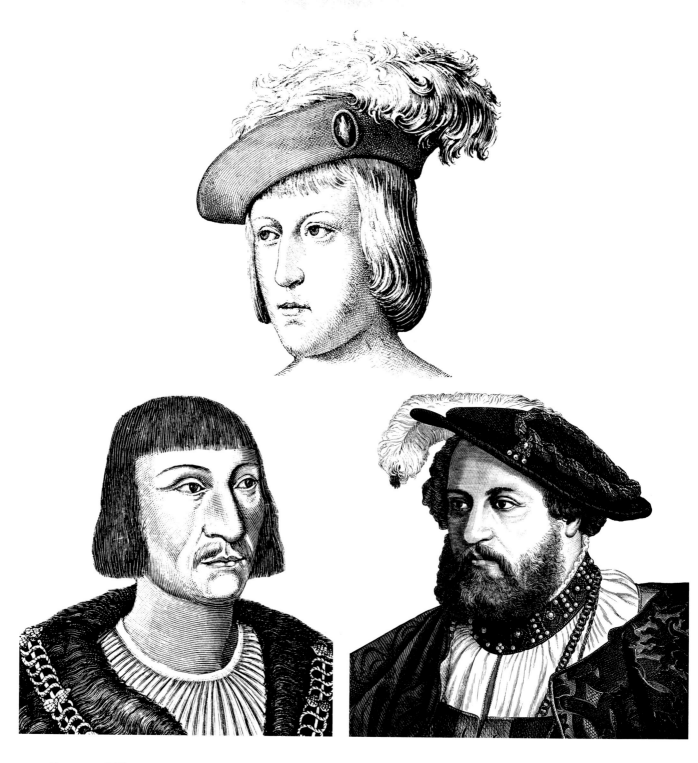

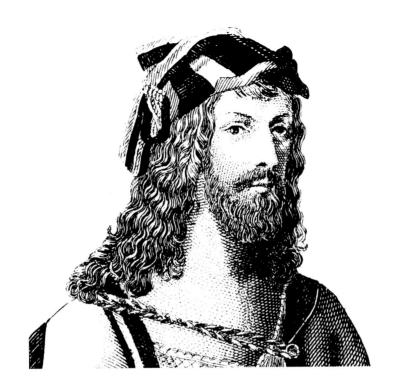

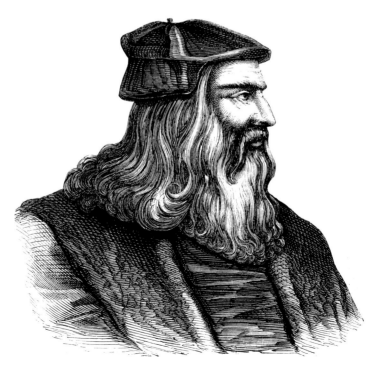

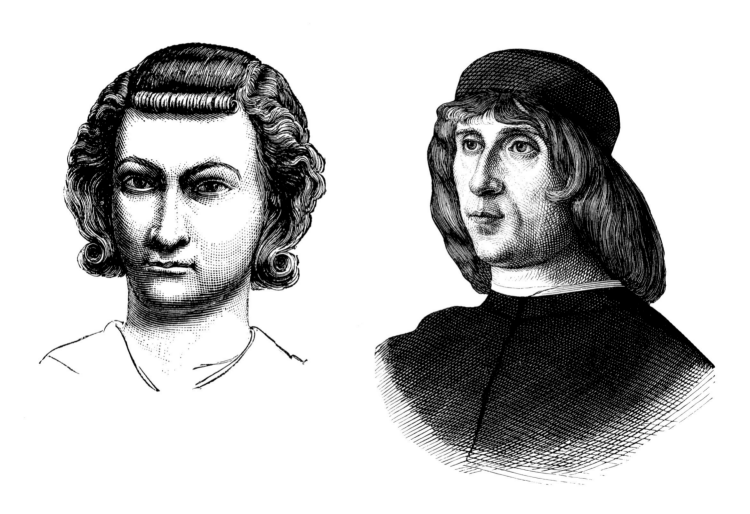

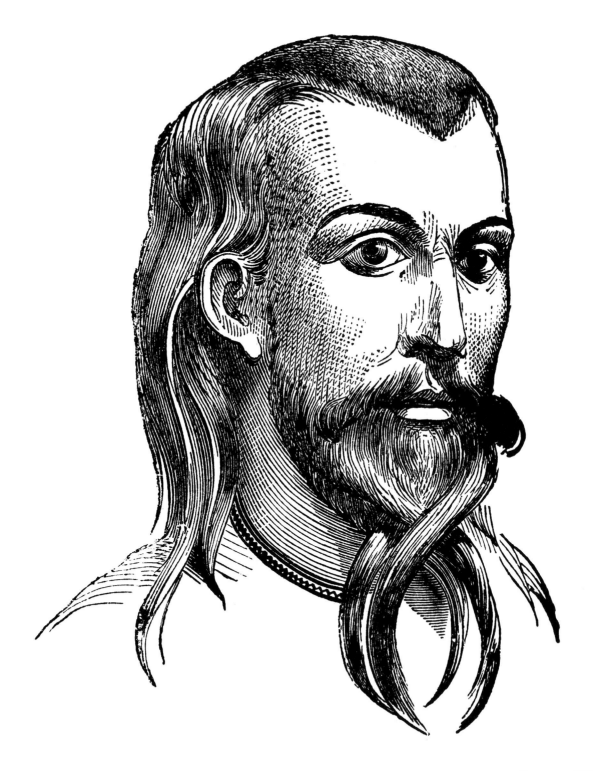

Europe, c. 1500   51

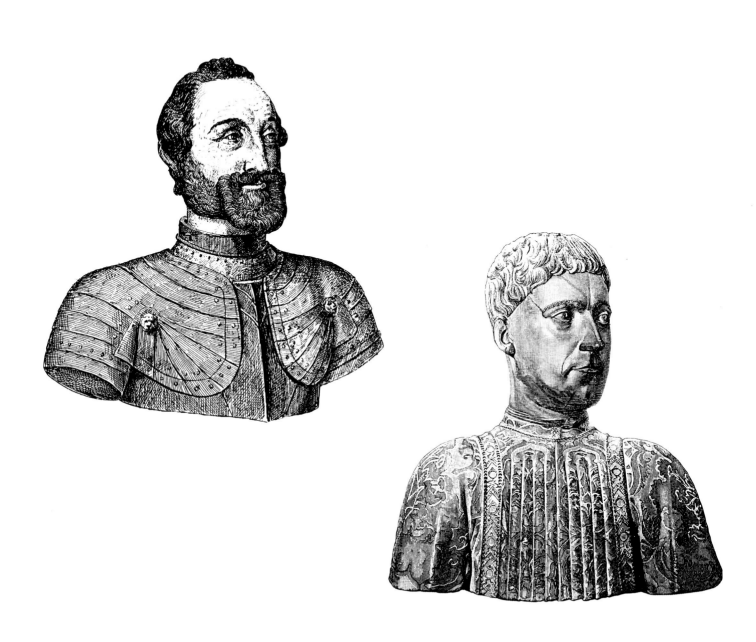

52   Military Hairstyles, c. 1500

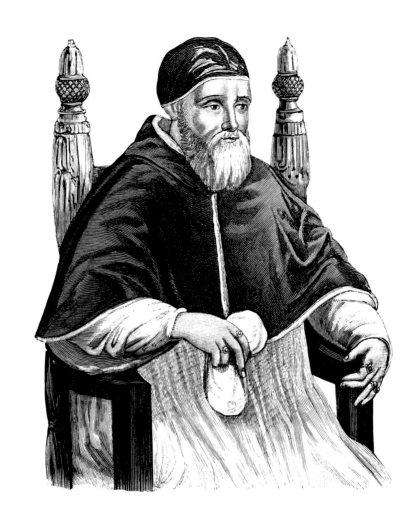

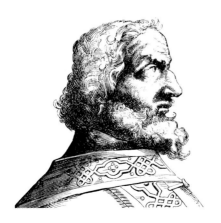

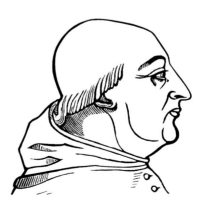

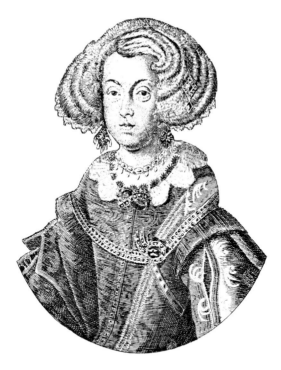

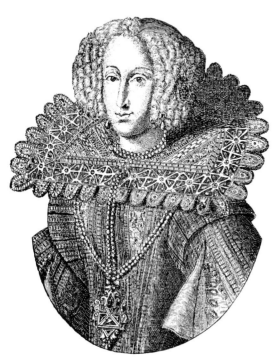

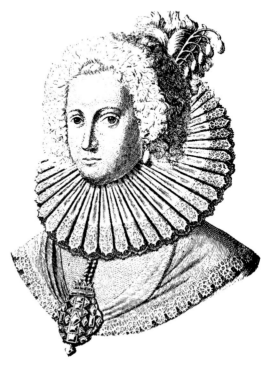

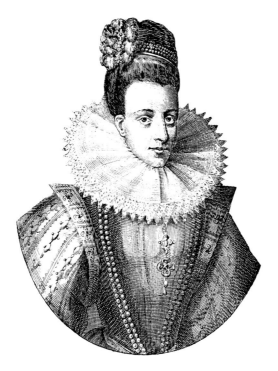

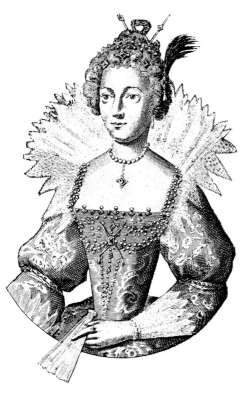

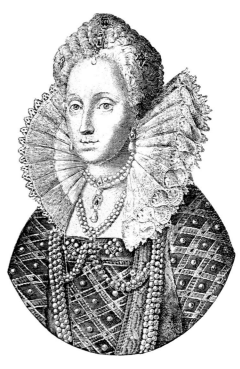

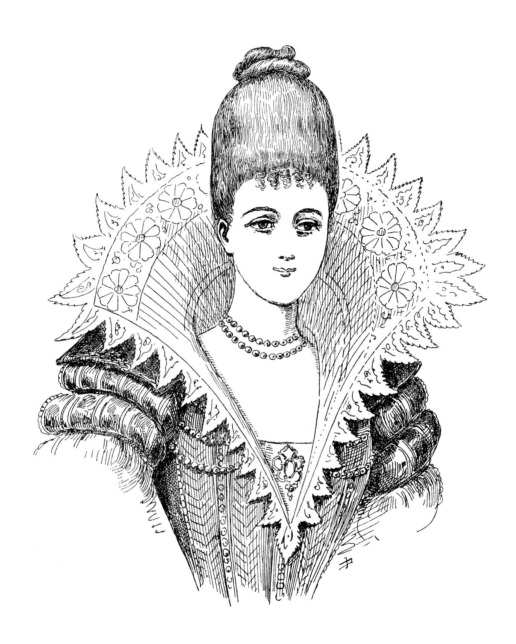

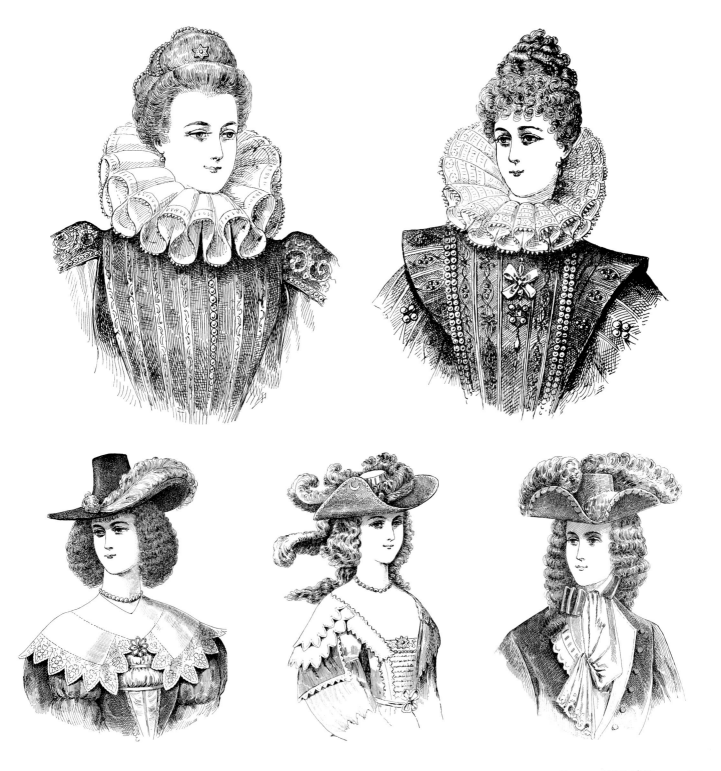

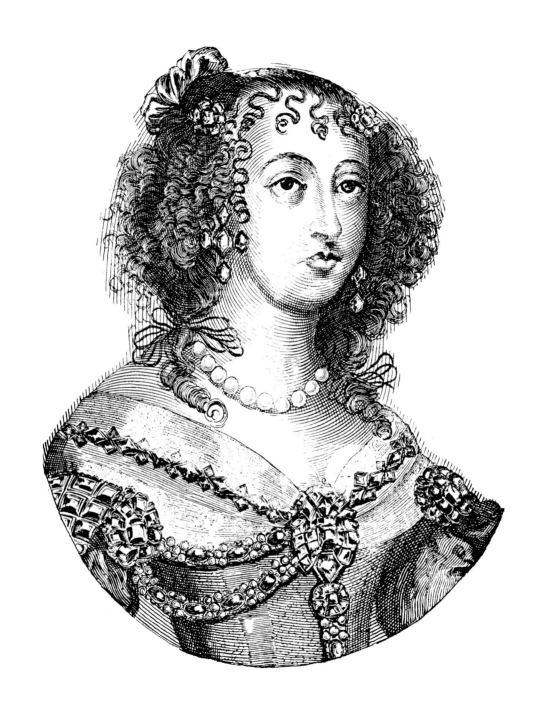

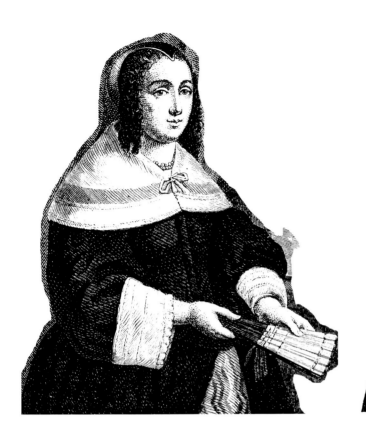
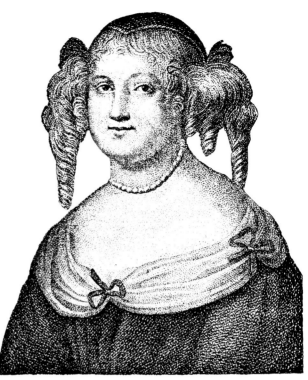
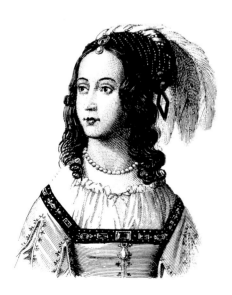
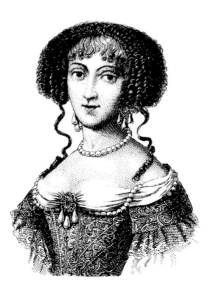
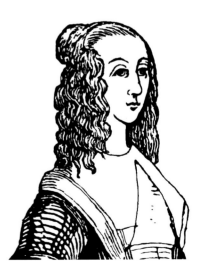

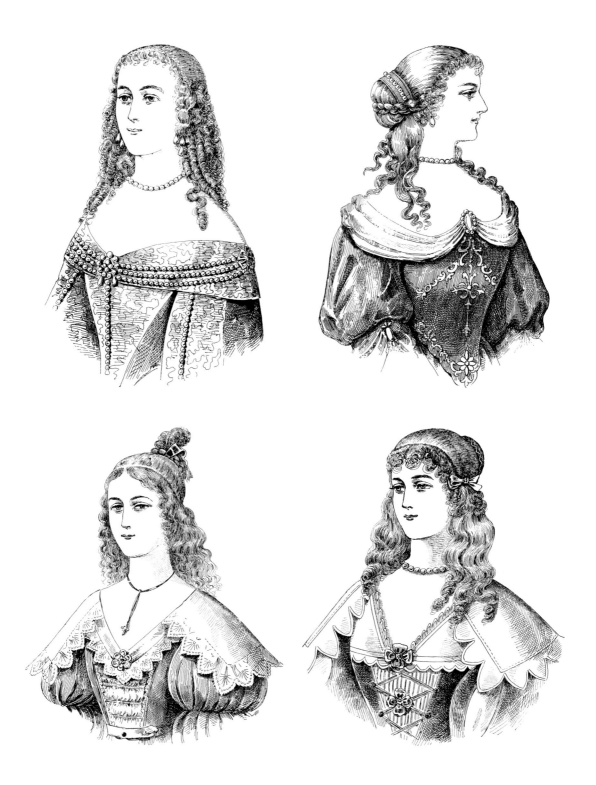

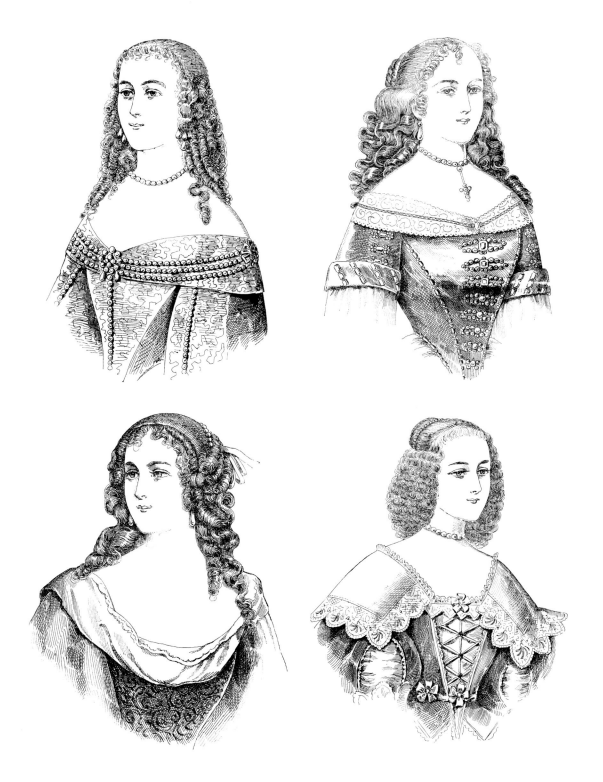

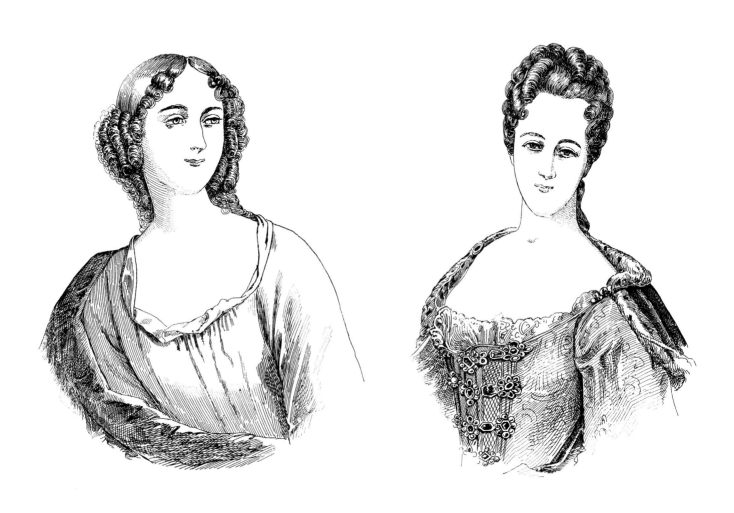

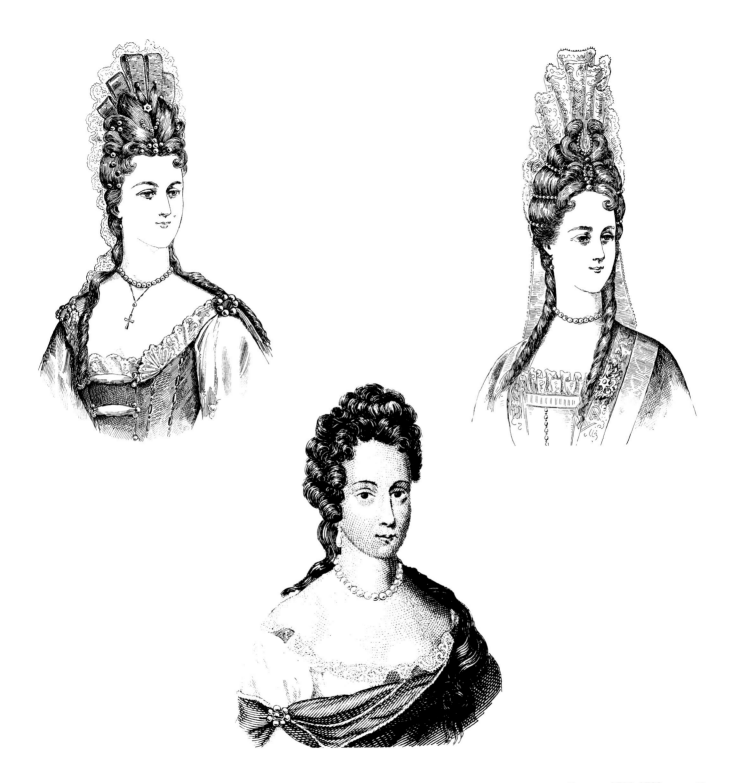

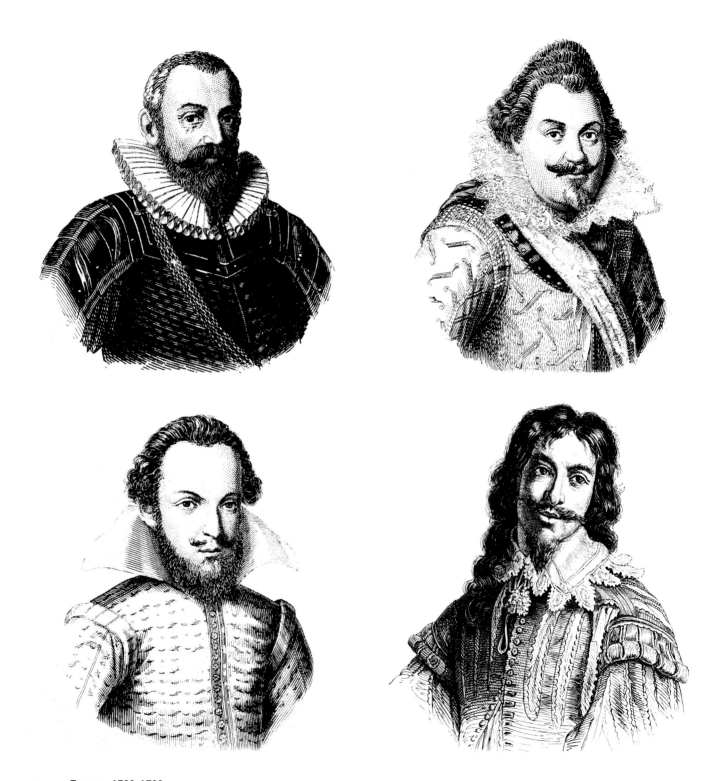

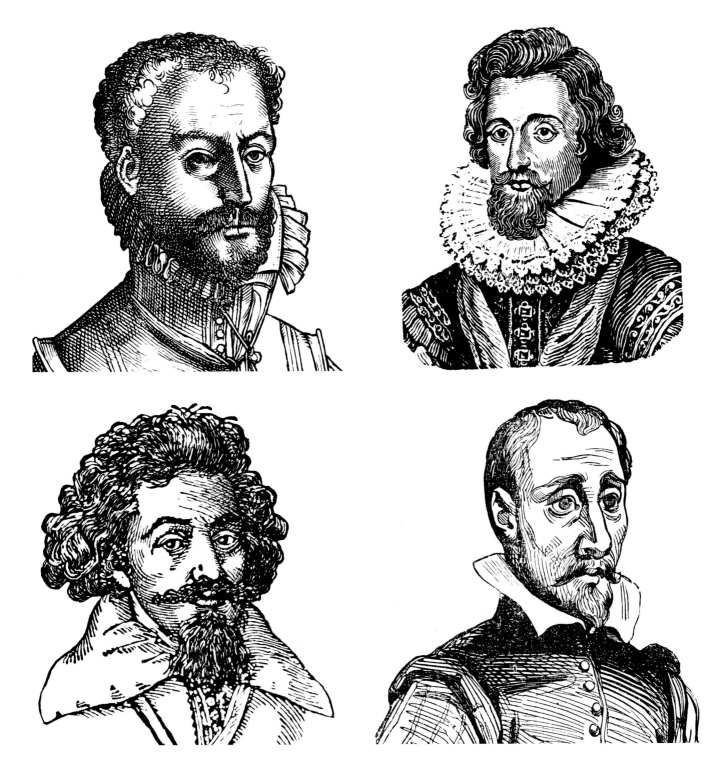

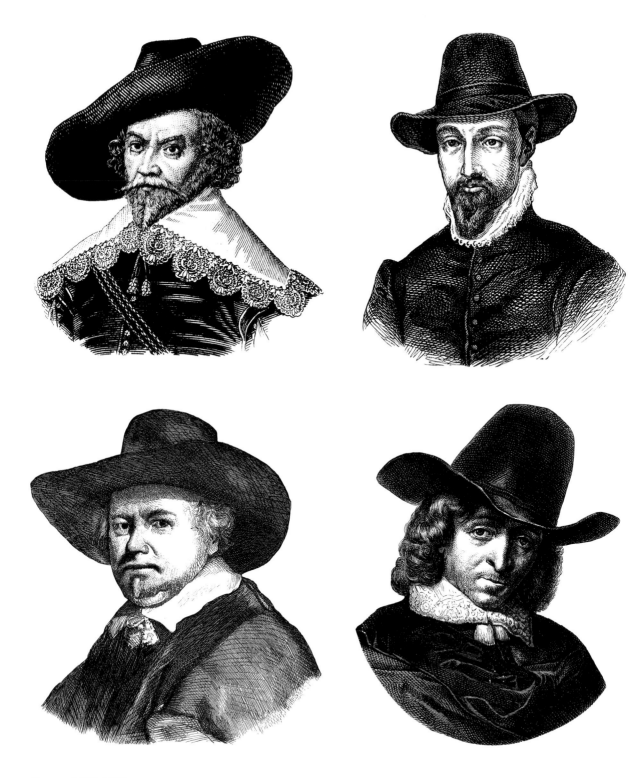

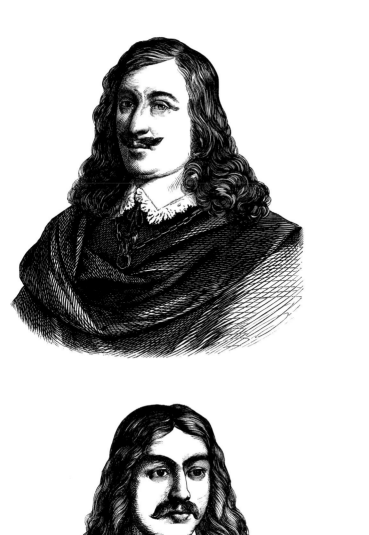

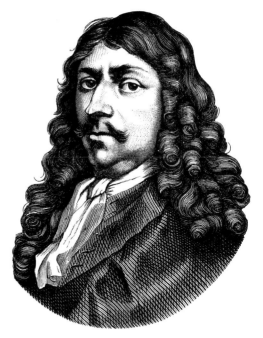

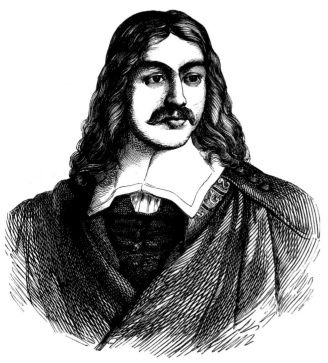

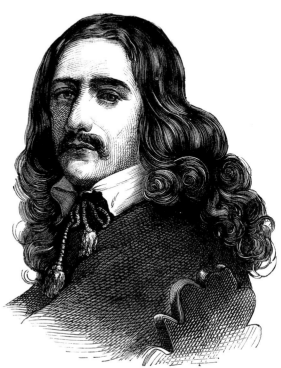

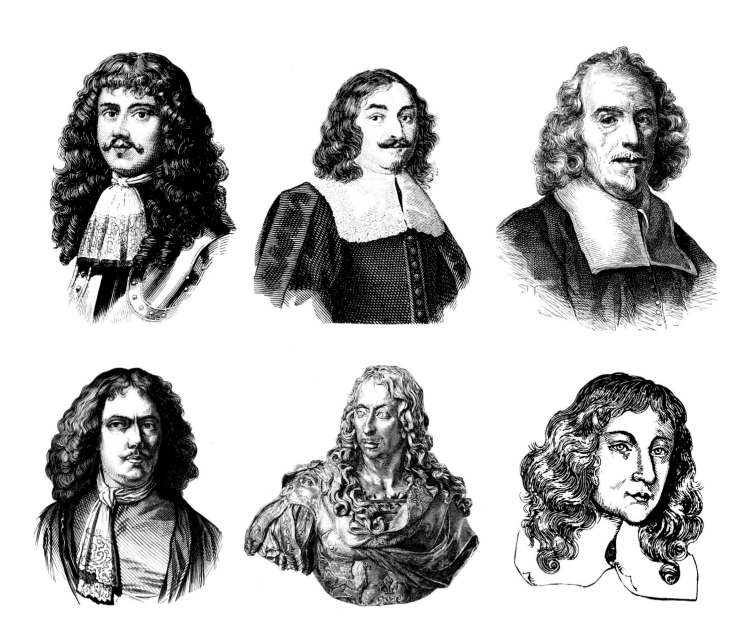

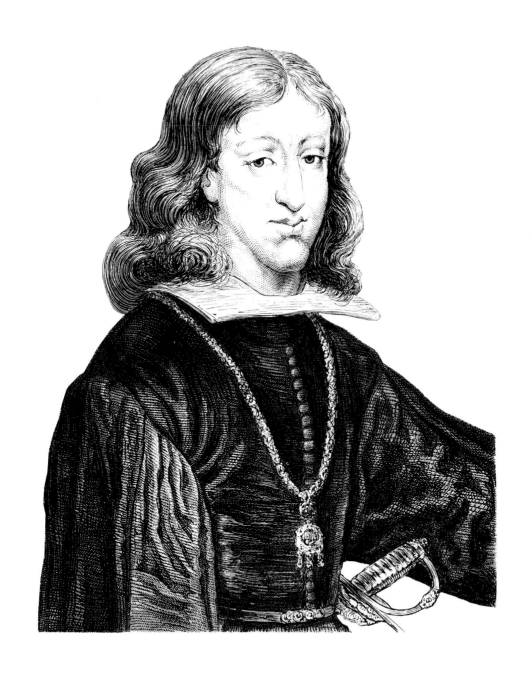

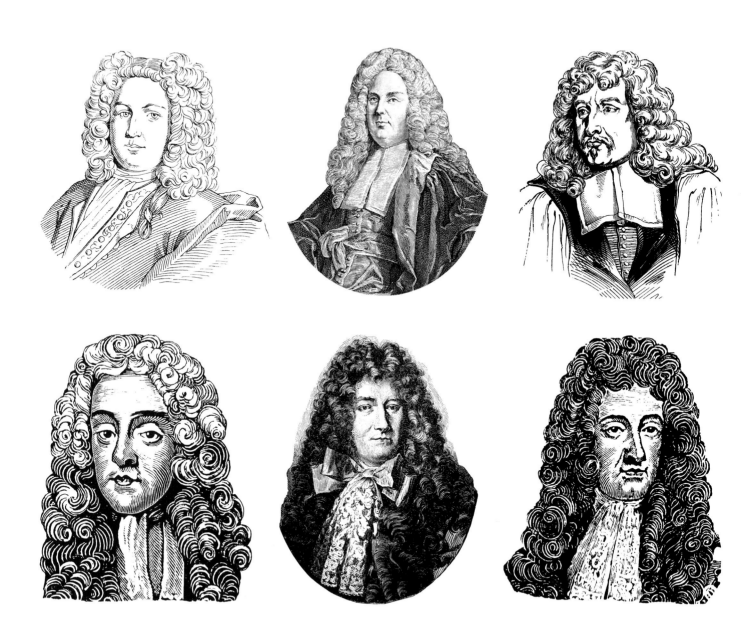

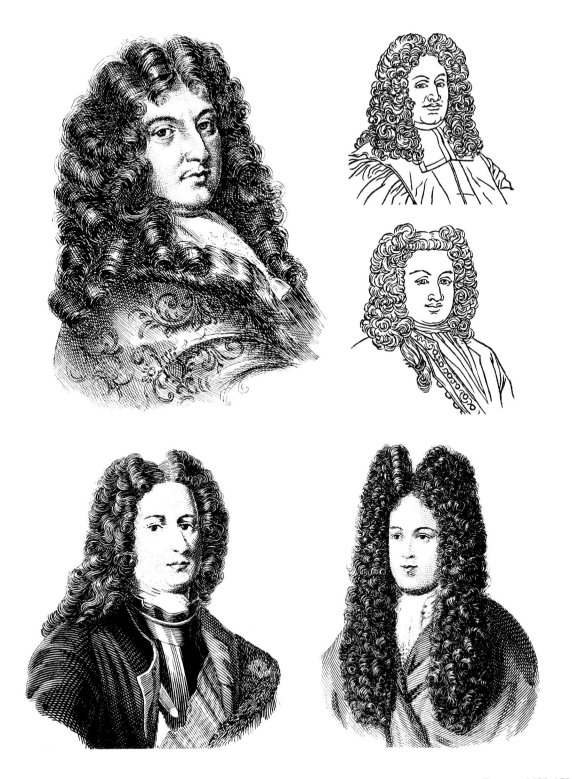

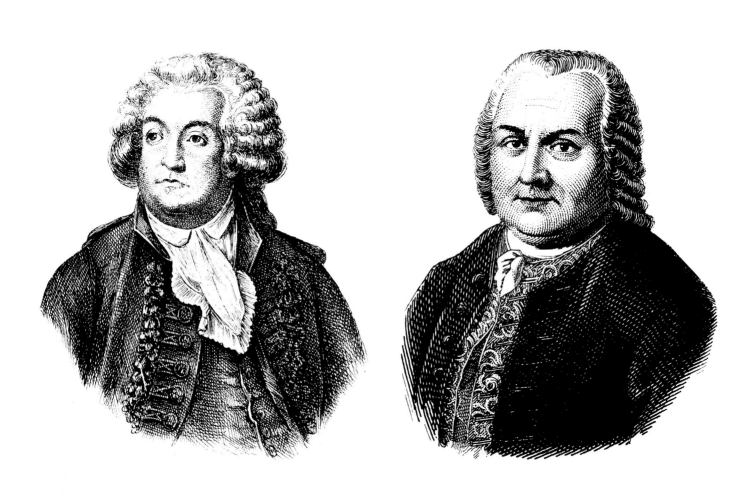

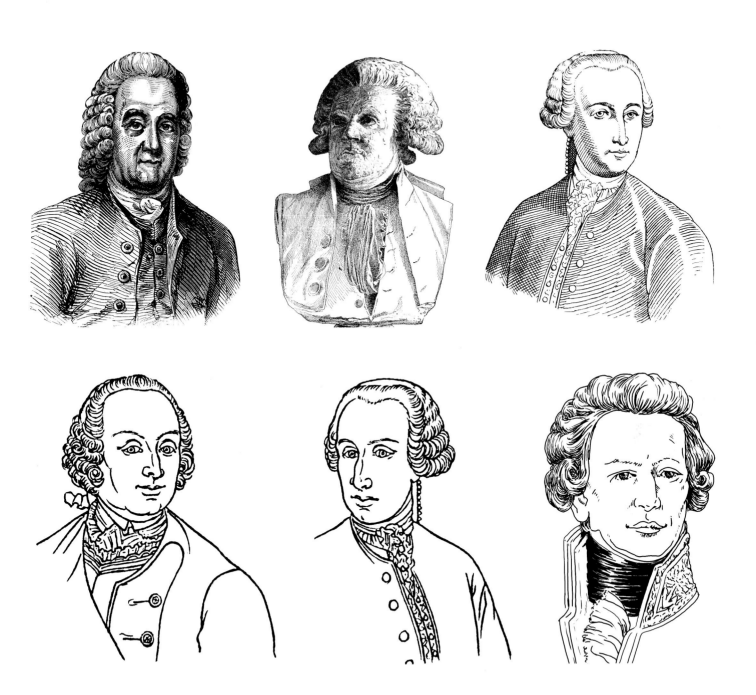

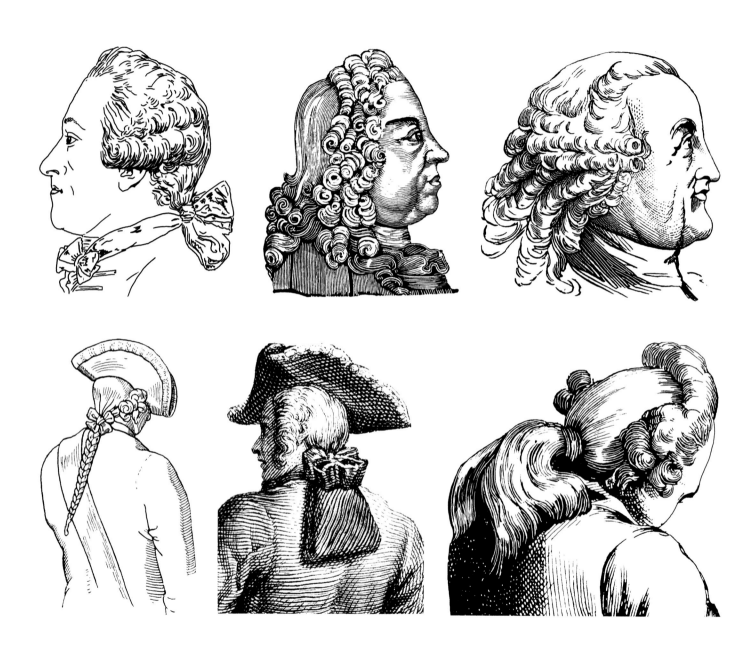

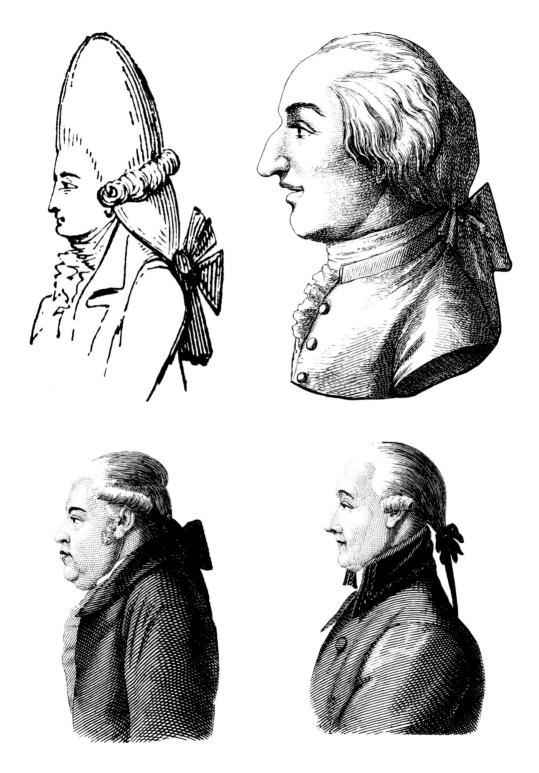

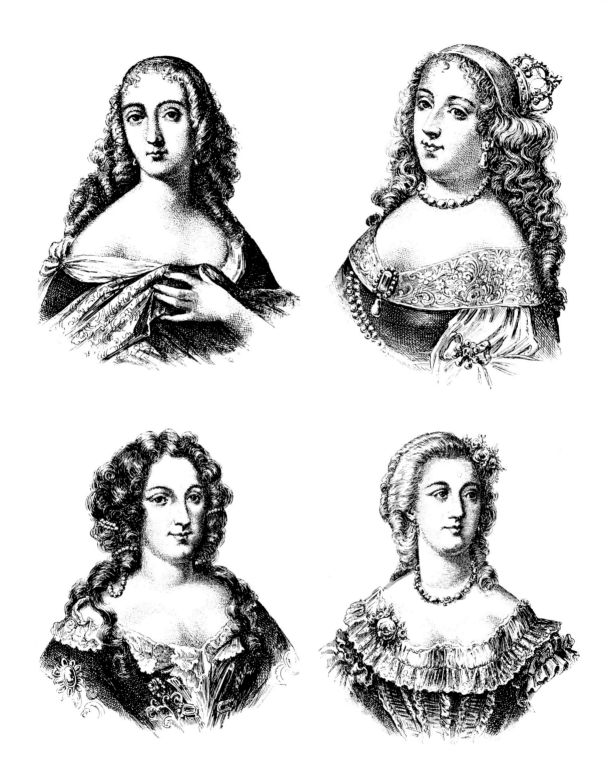

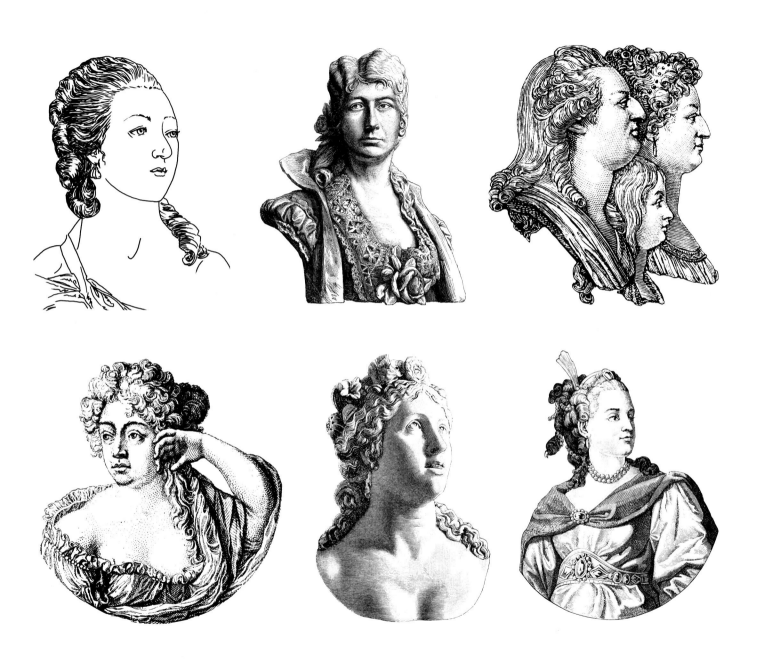

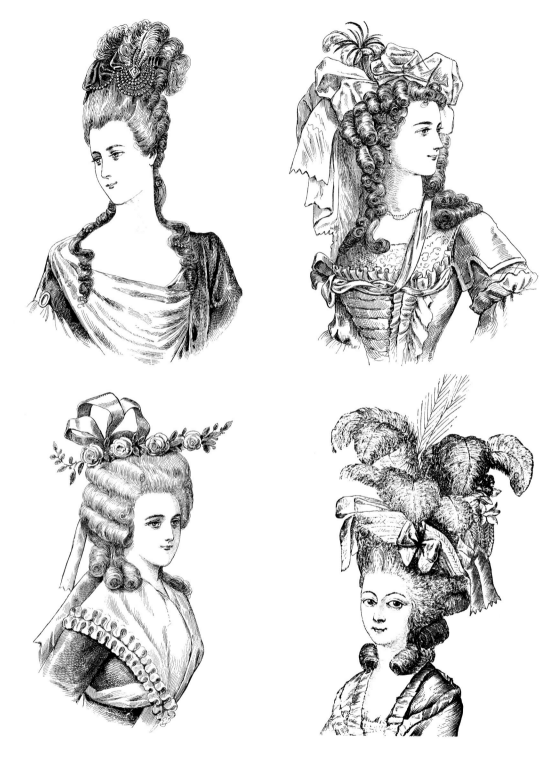

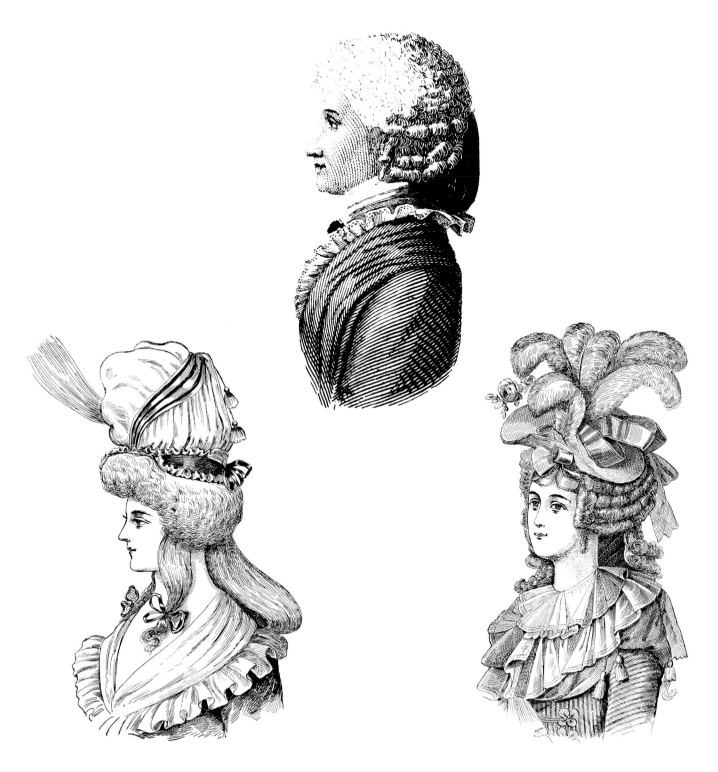

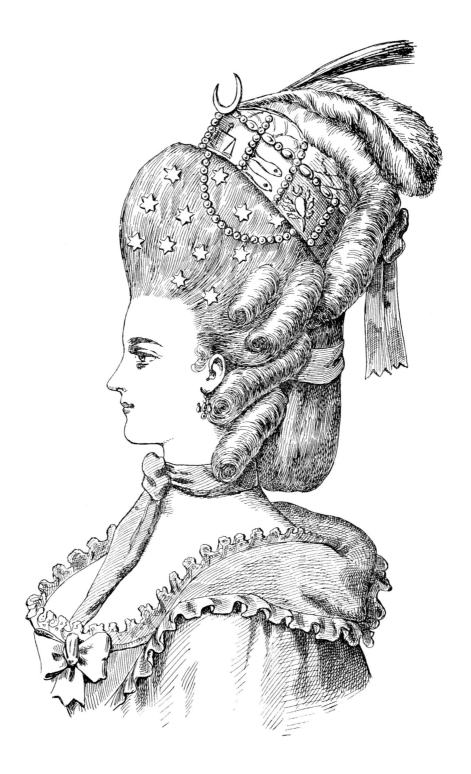

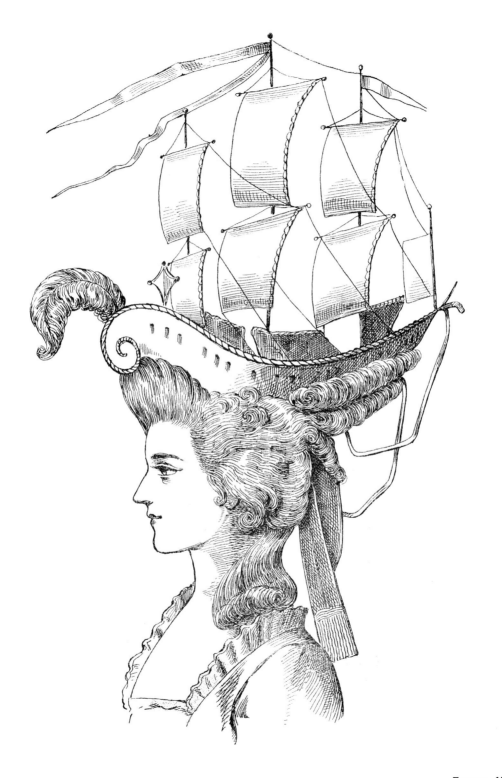

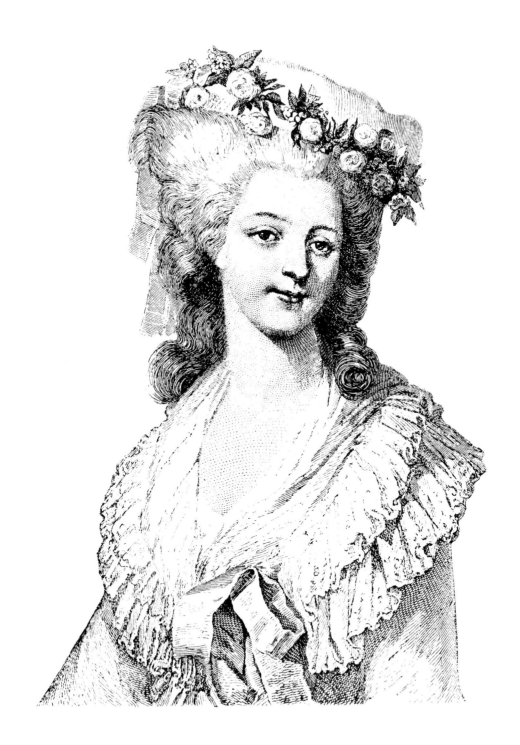

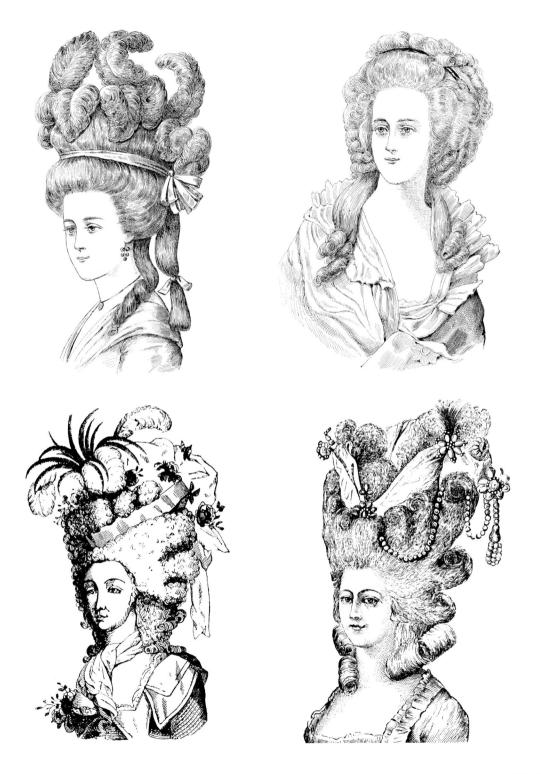

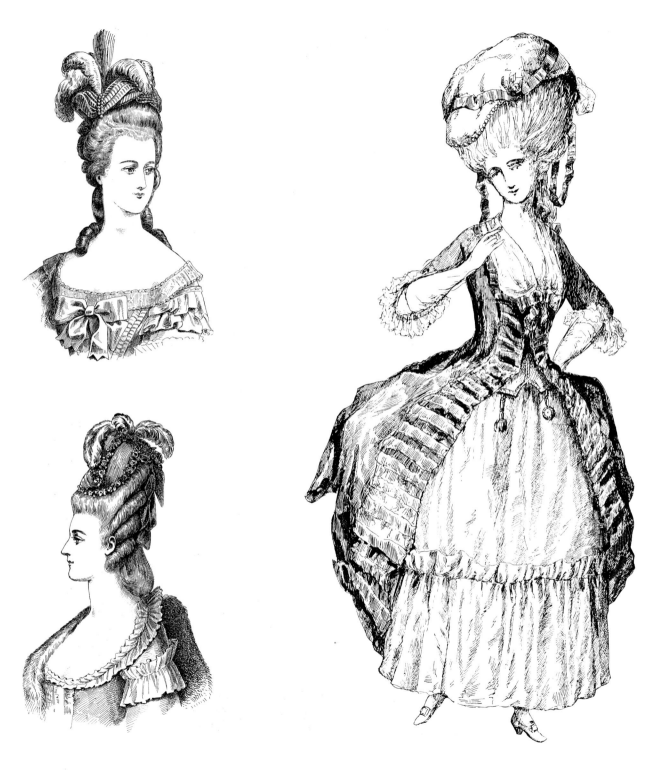

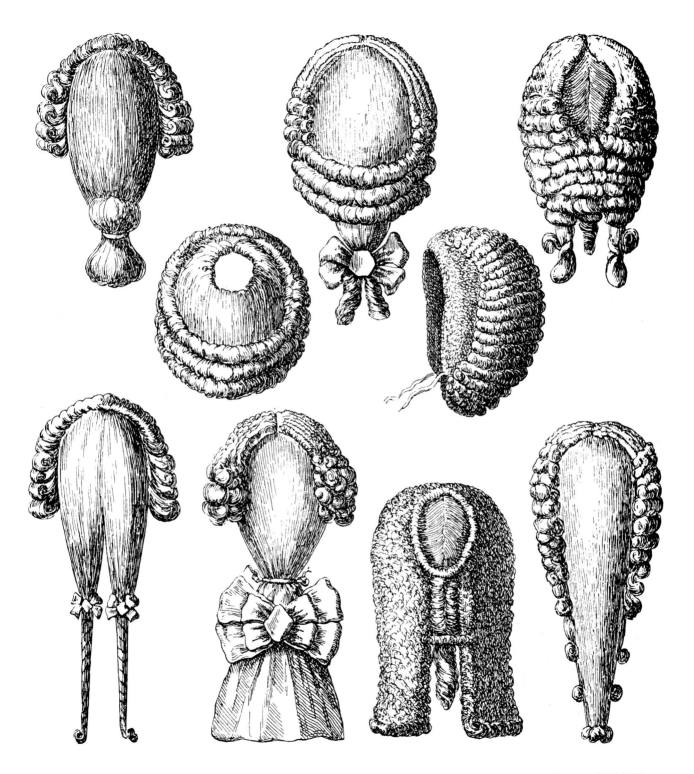

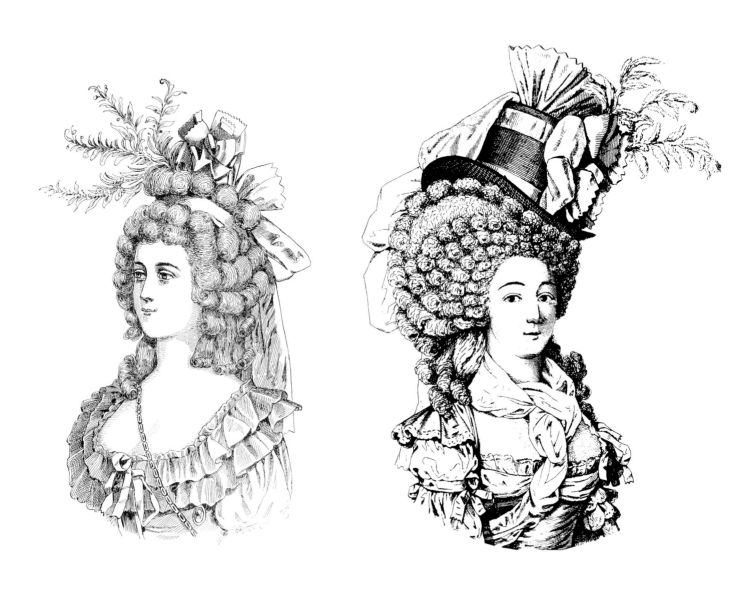

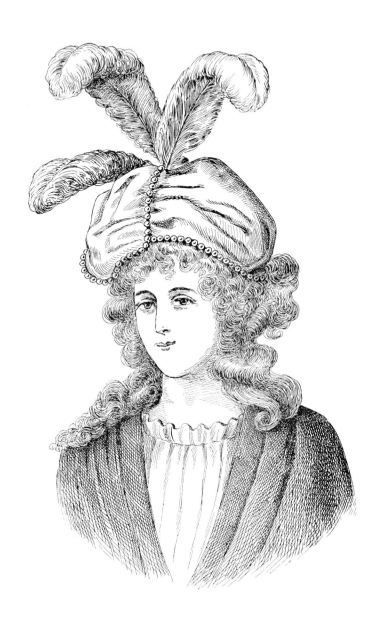

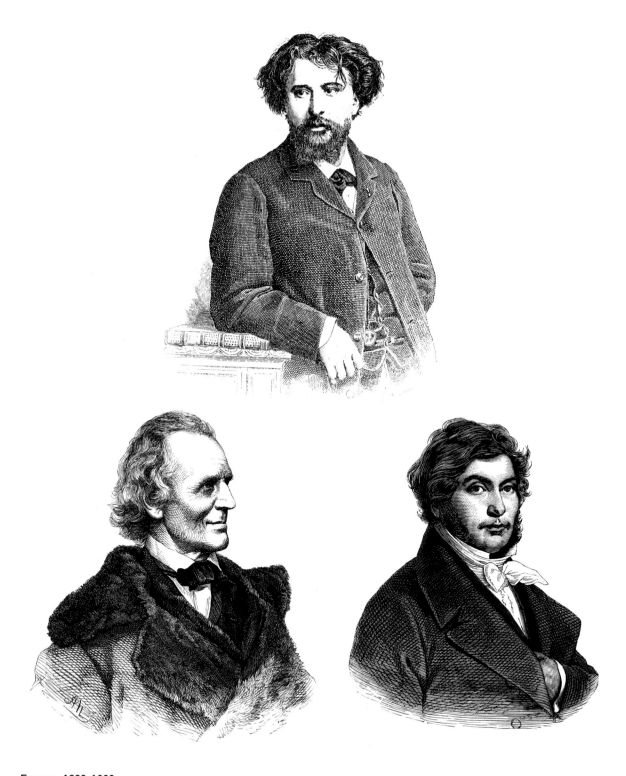

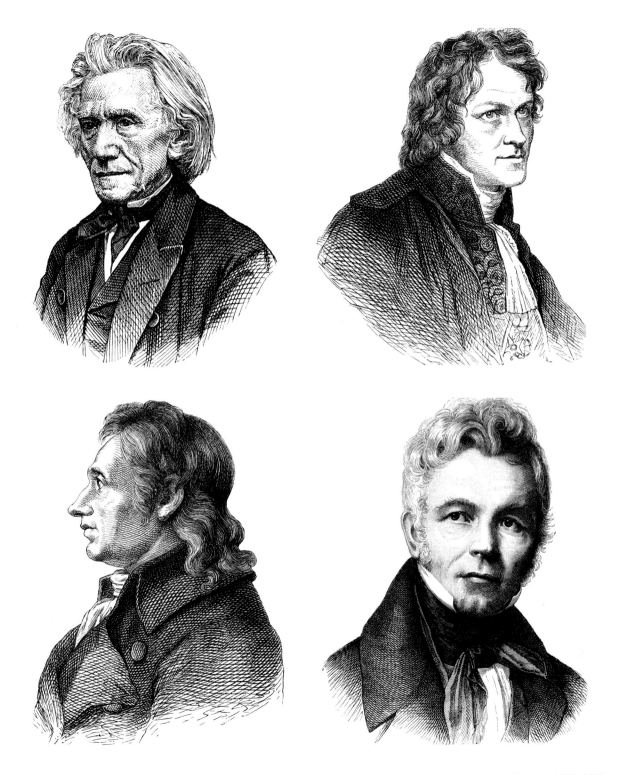

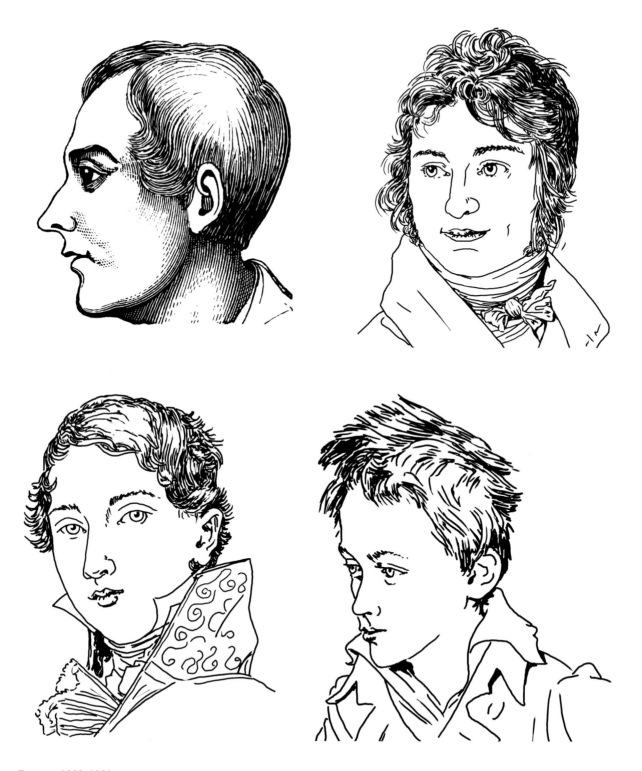

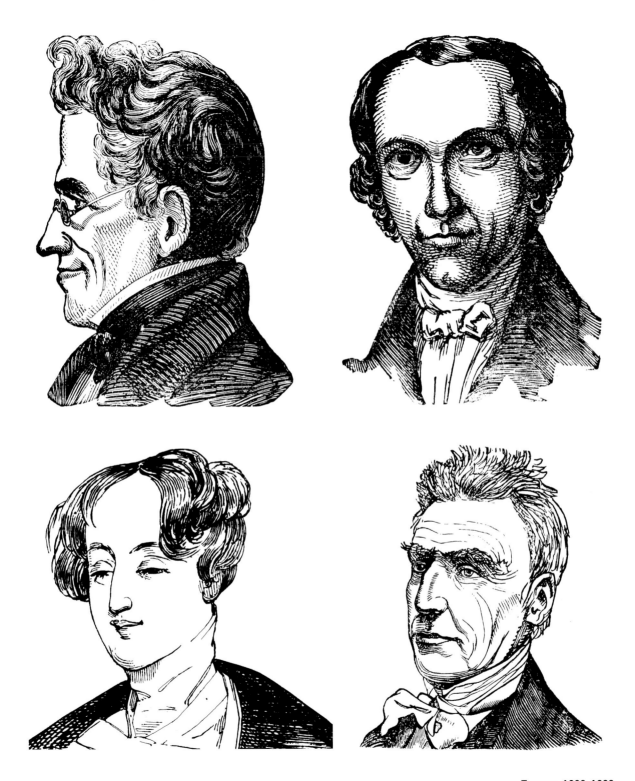

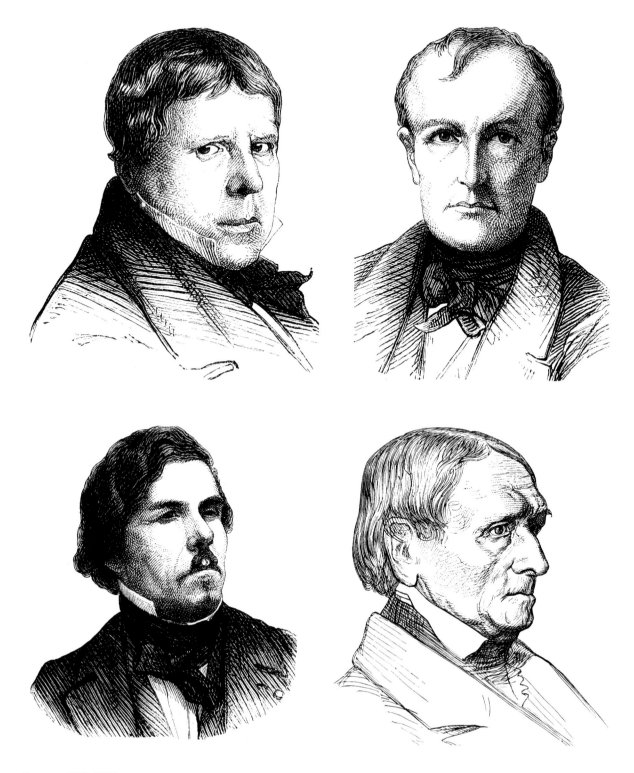

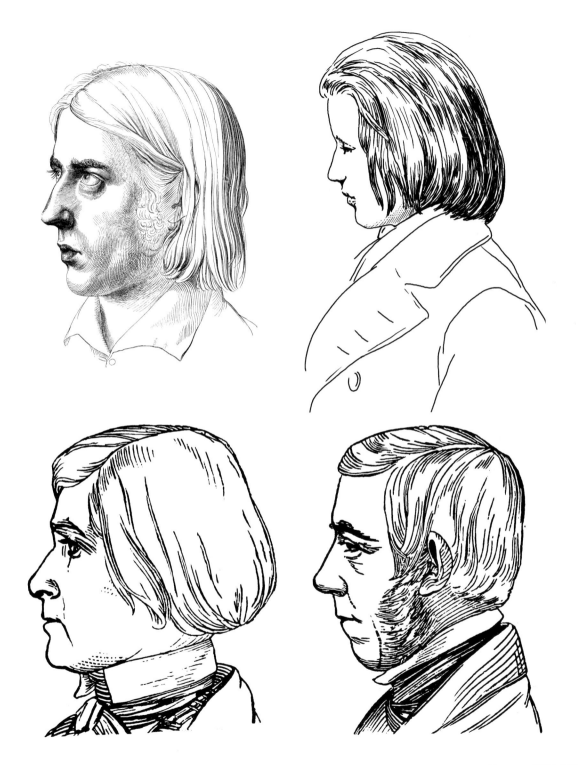

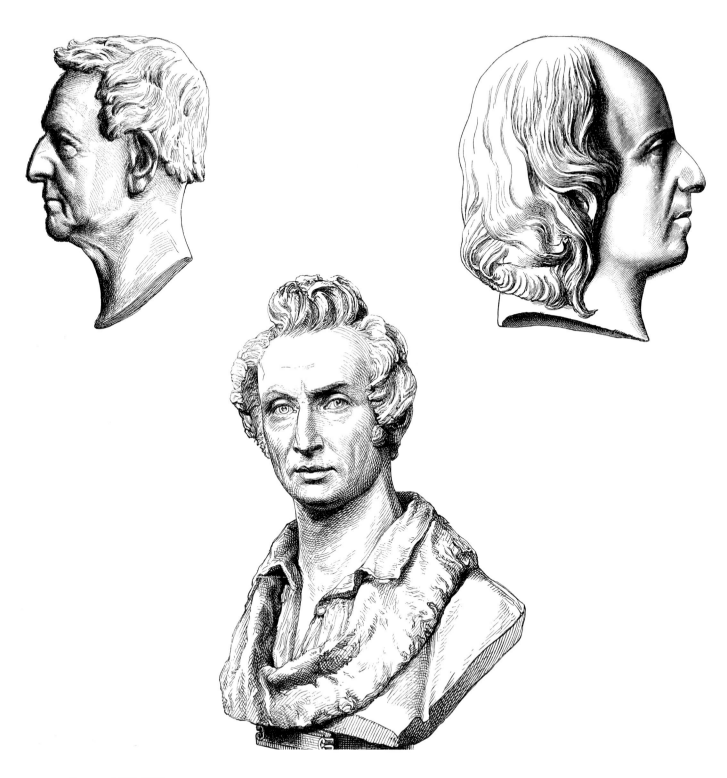

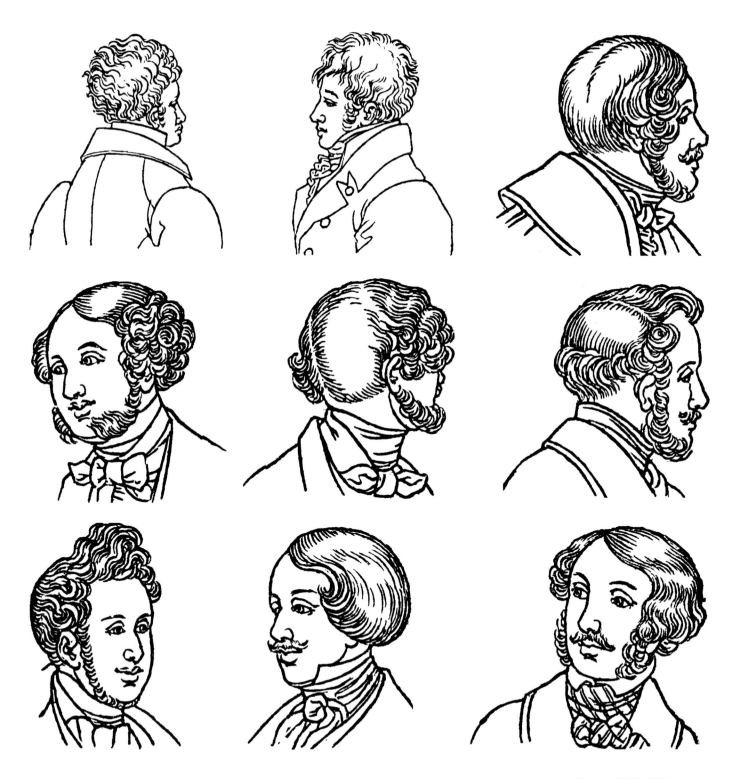

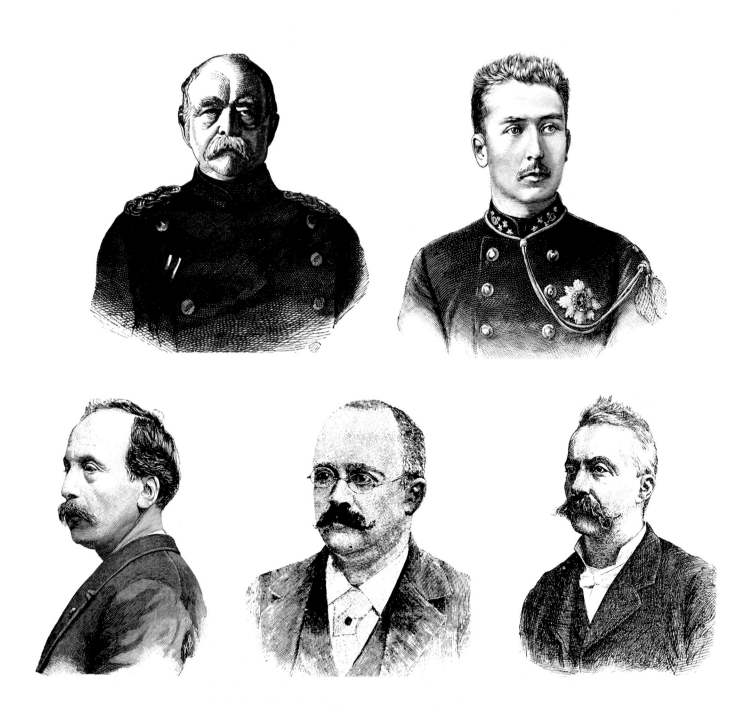

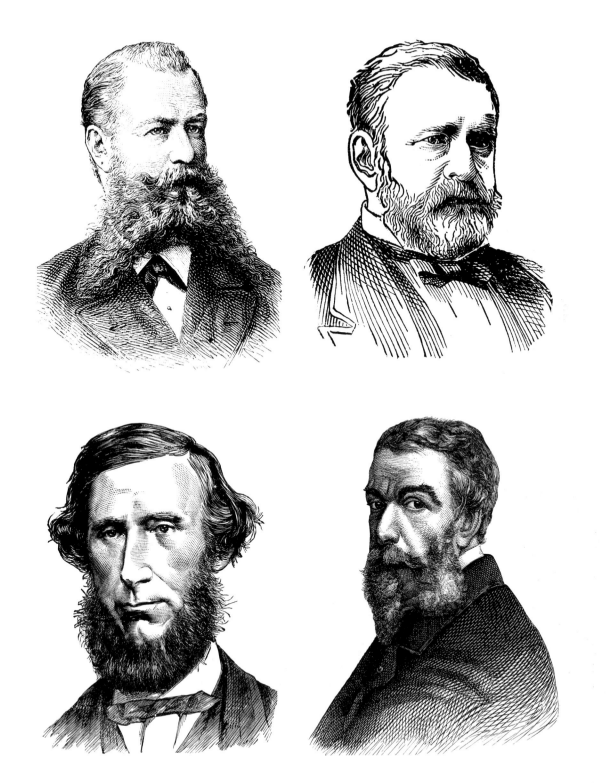

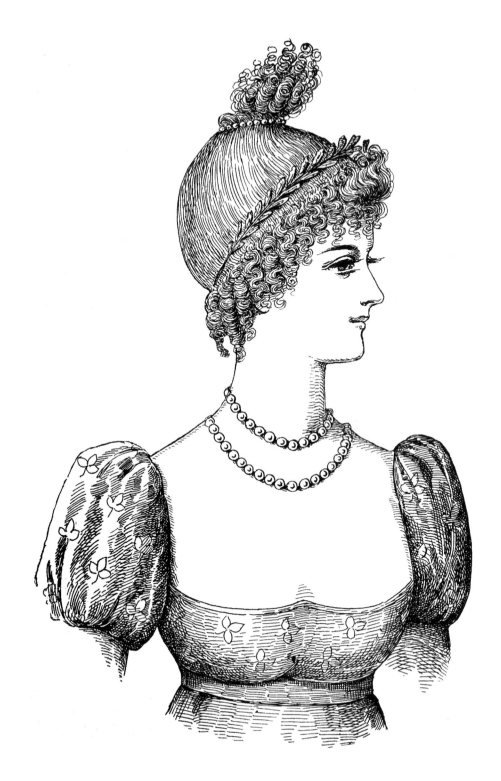

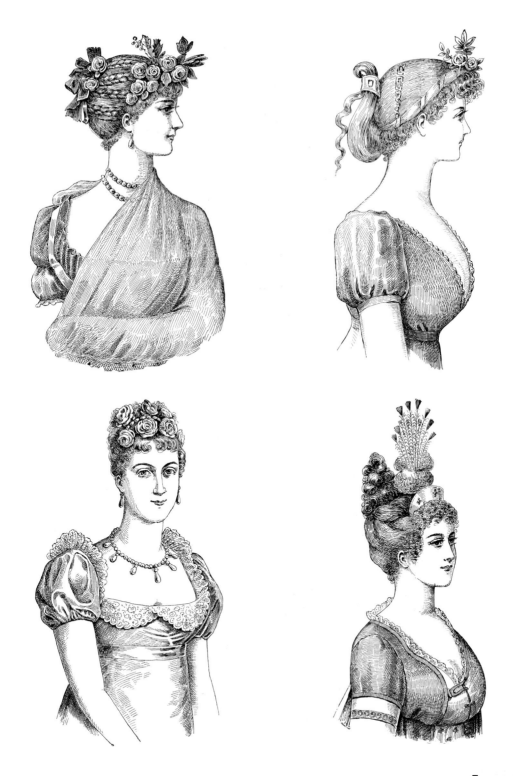

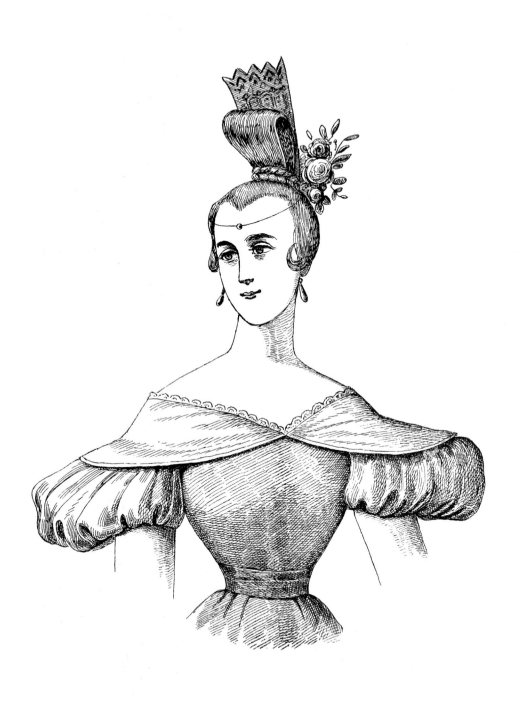

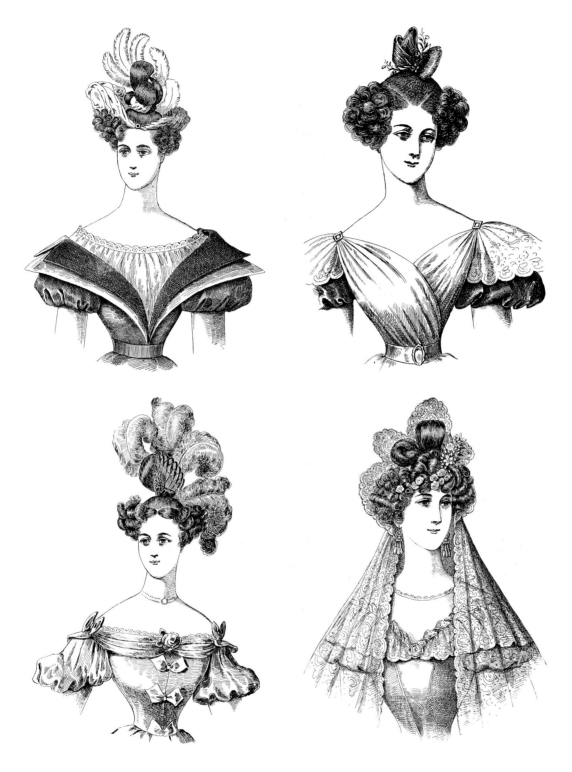

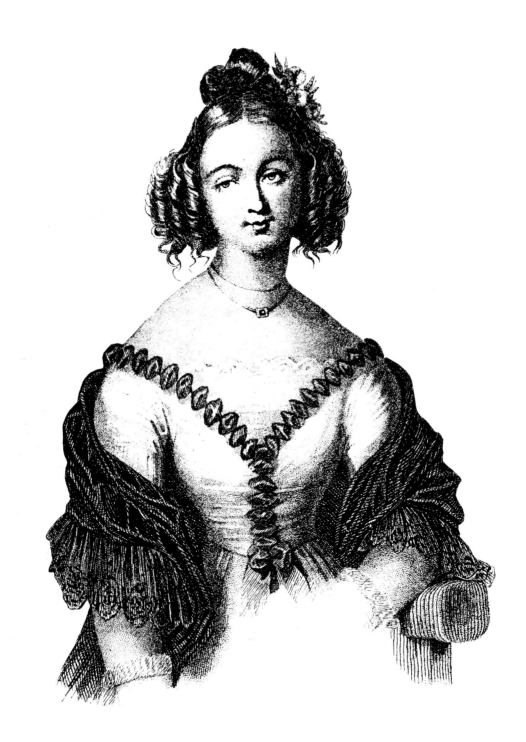

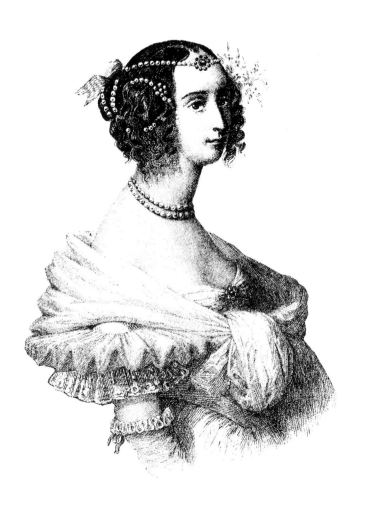
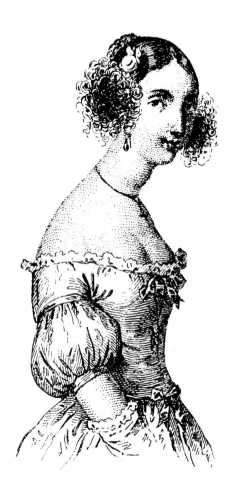

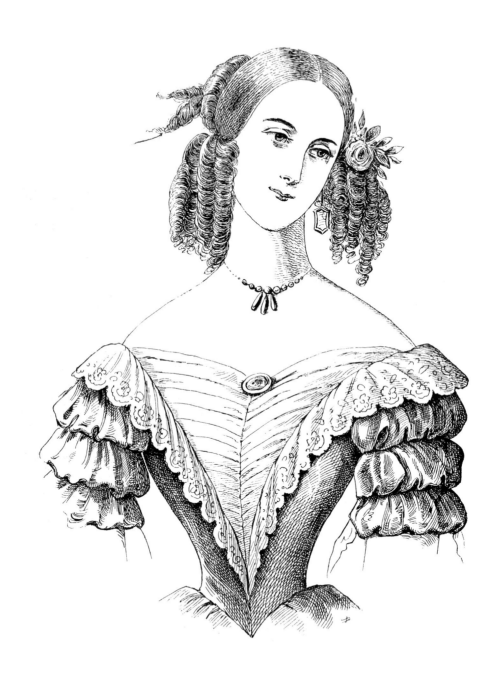

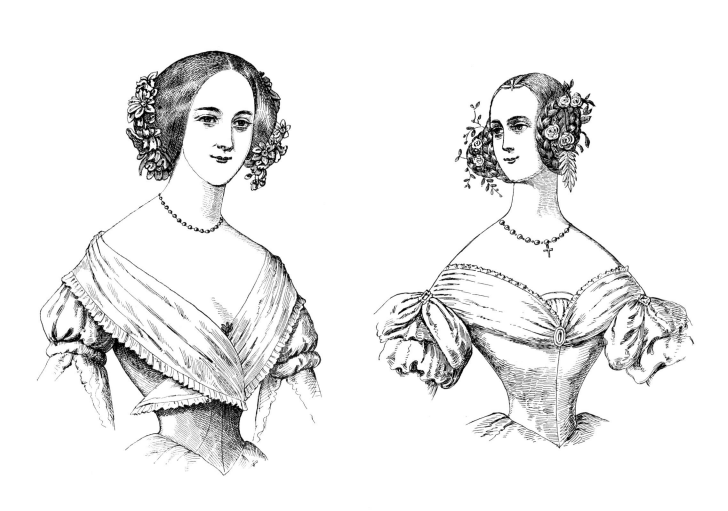

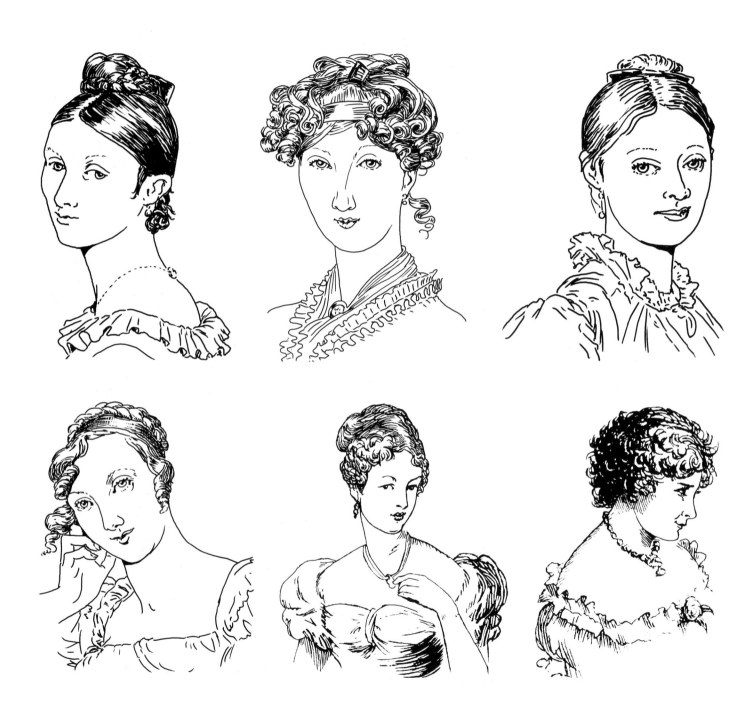

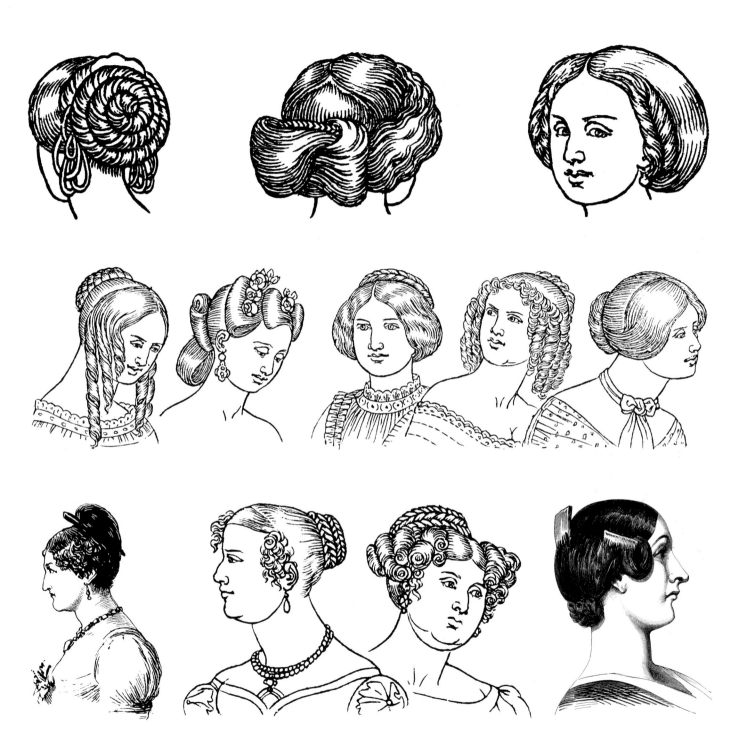

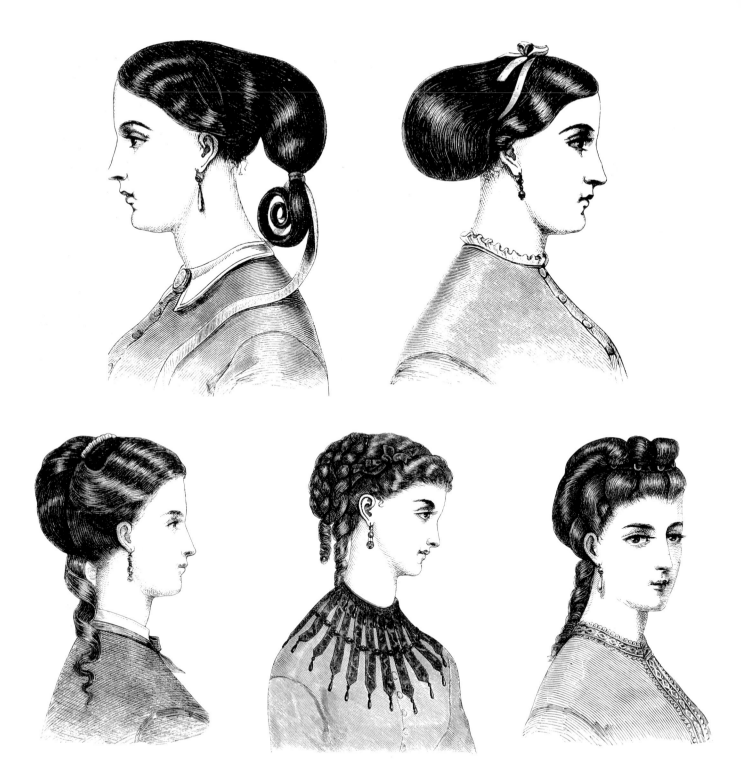

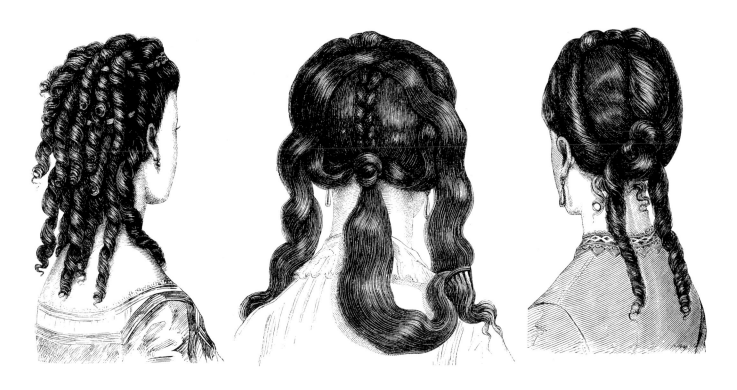

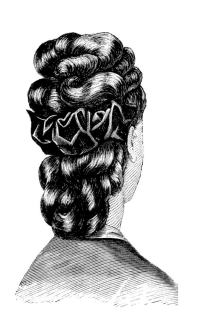

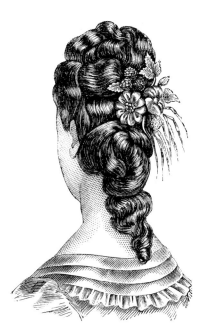

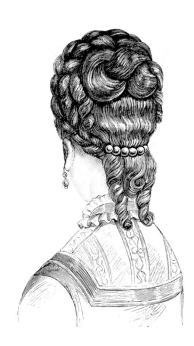

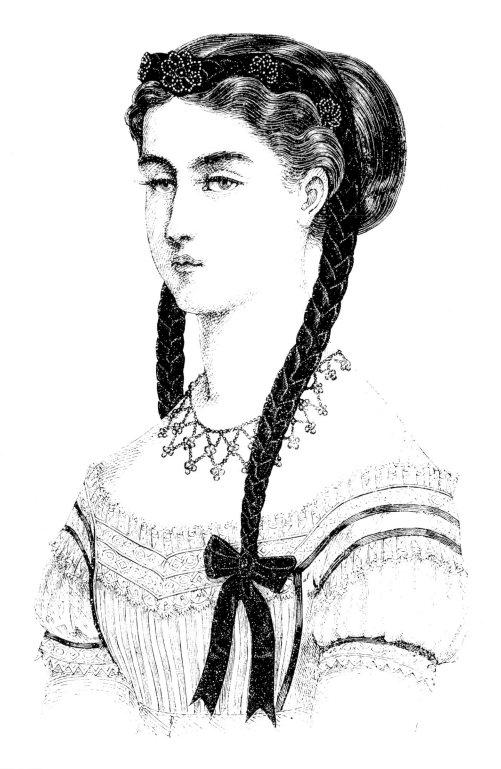

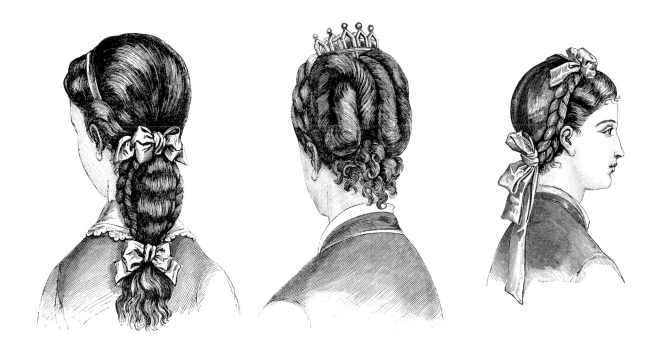

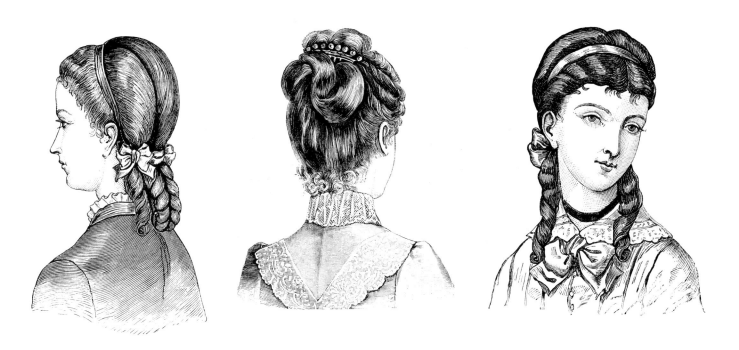

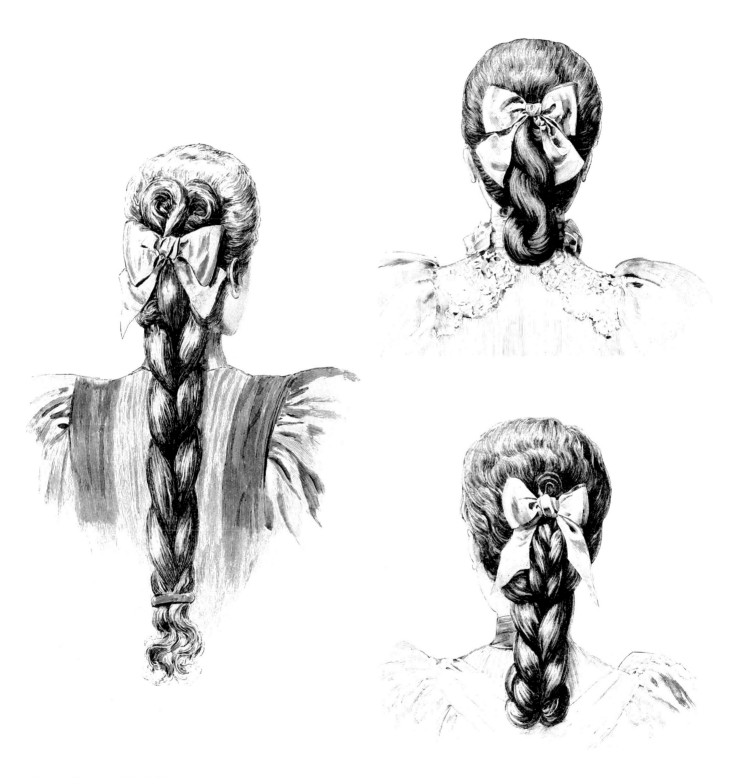

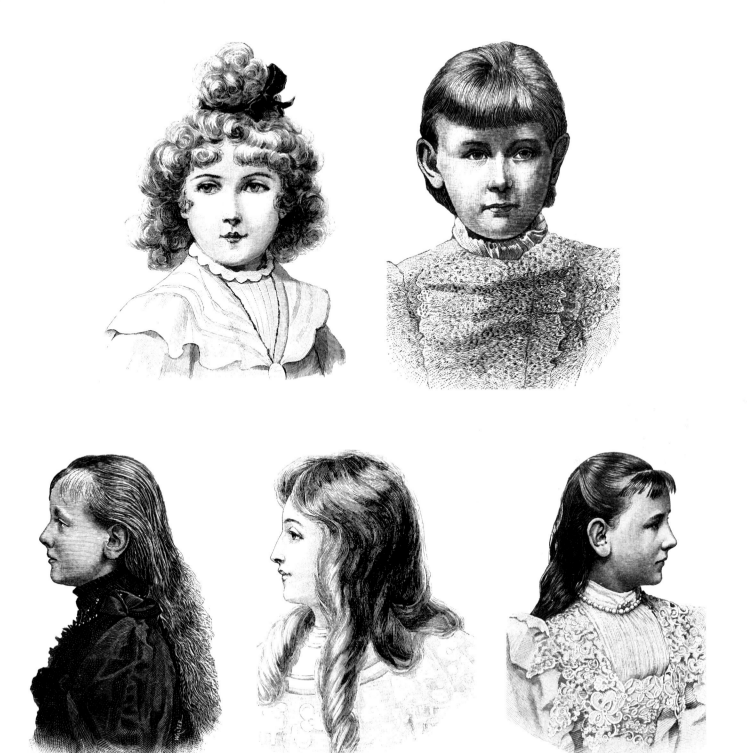

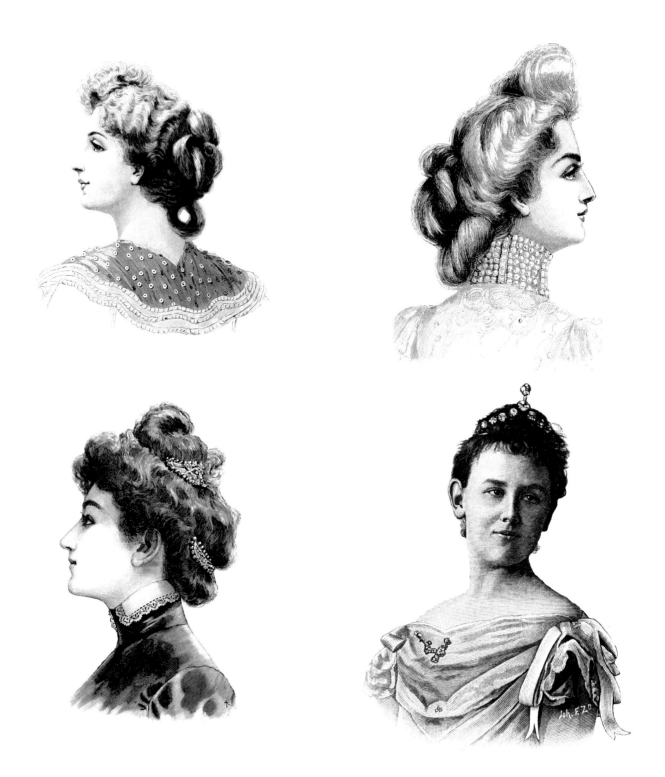

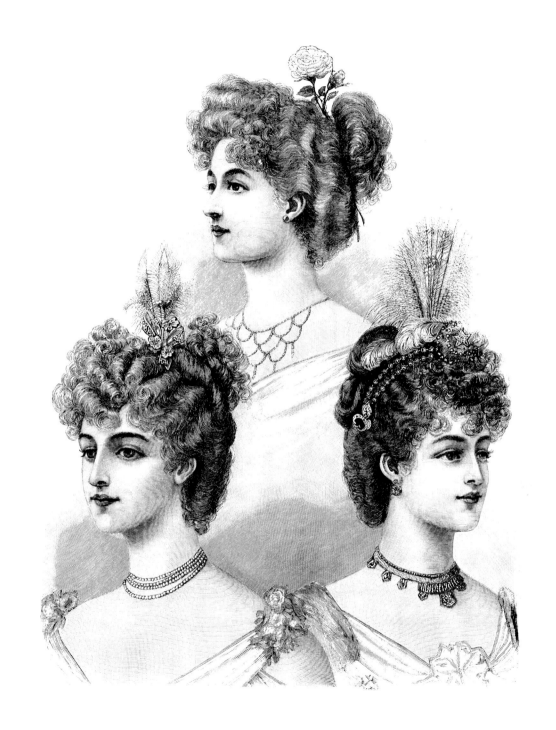

WESTERN HAIRSTYLES
OF THE 20TH CENTURY

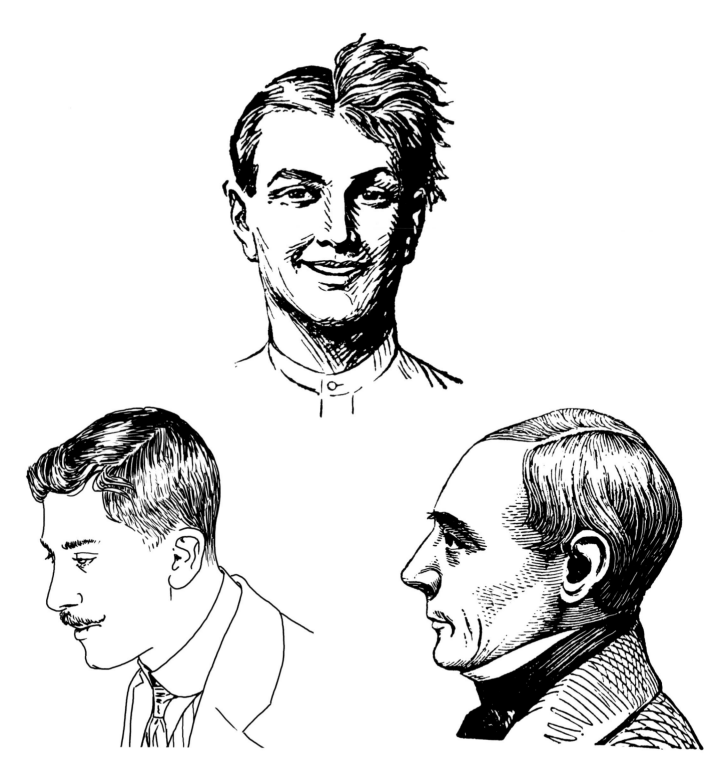

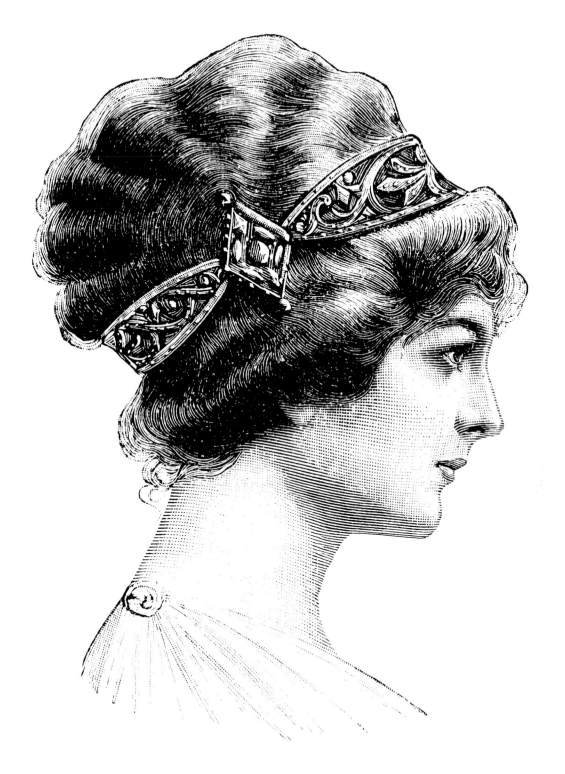

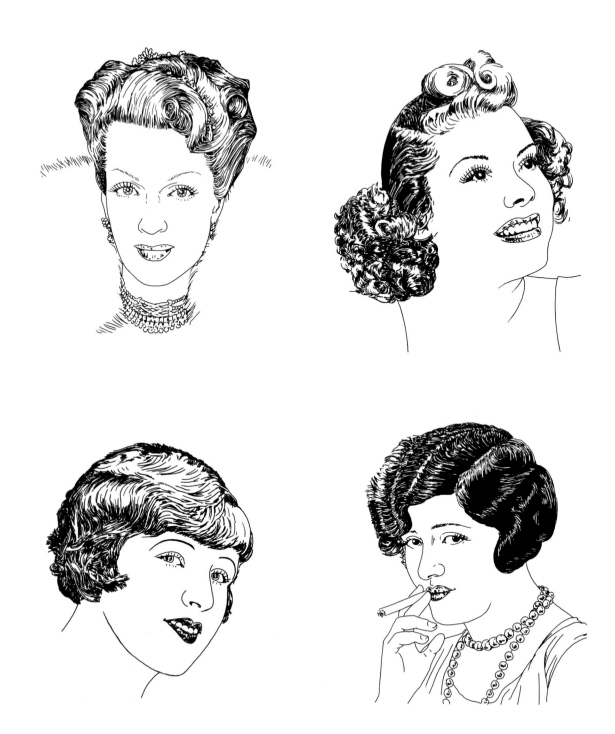

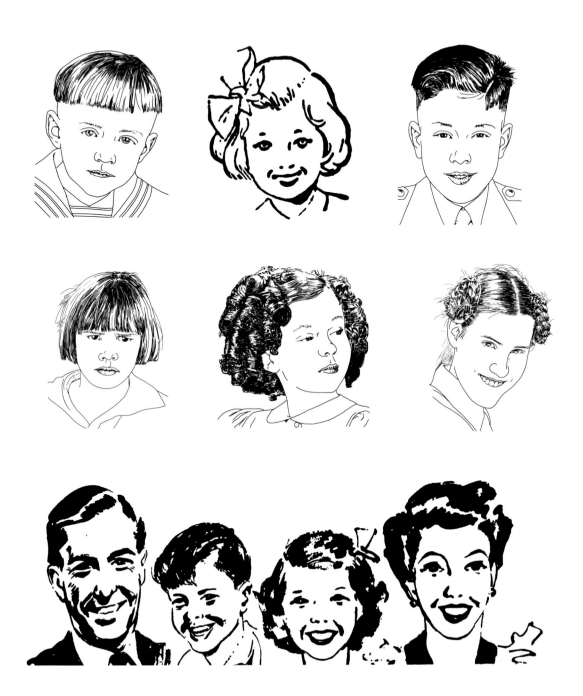

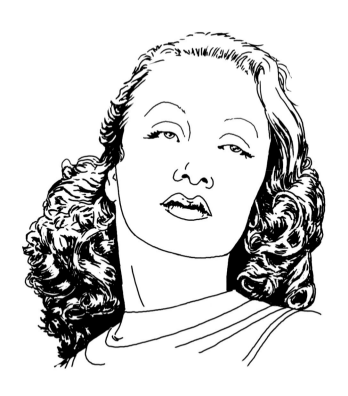

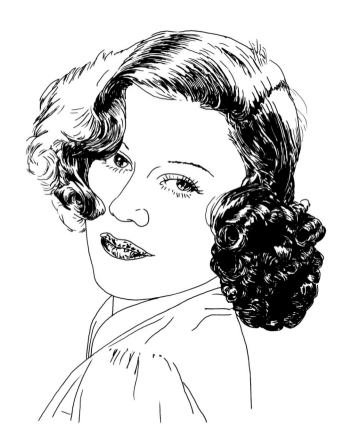

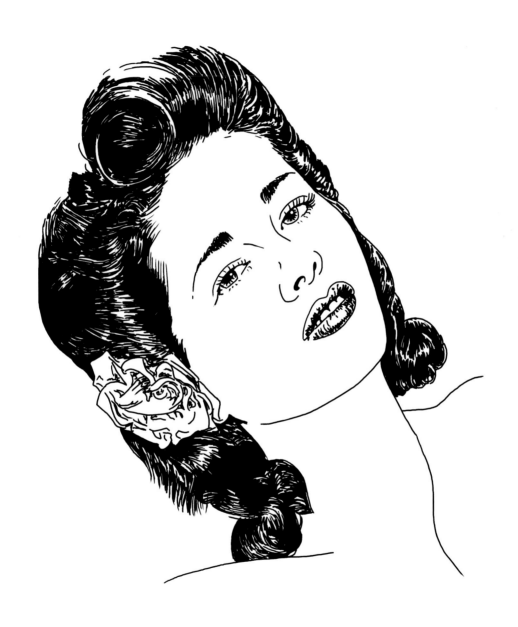

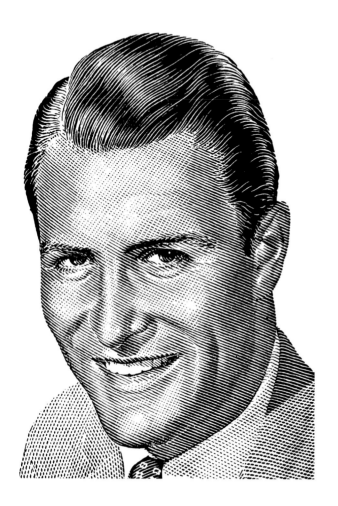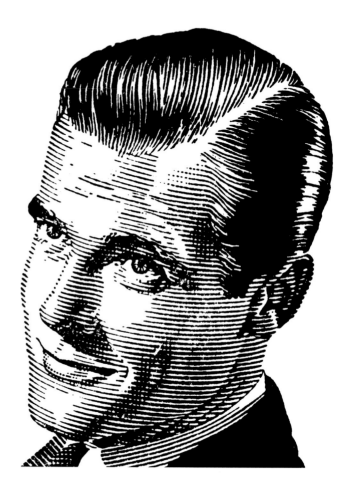

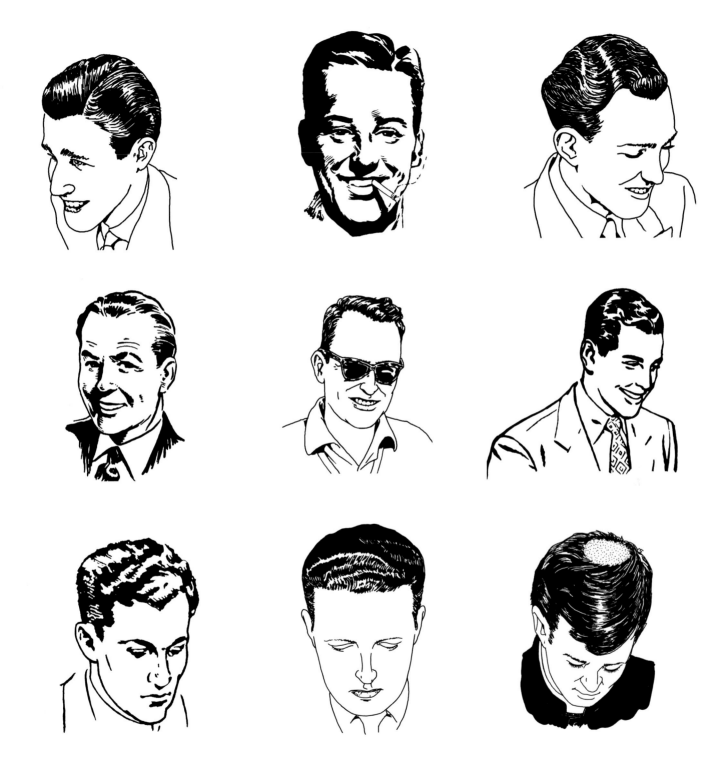

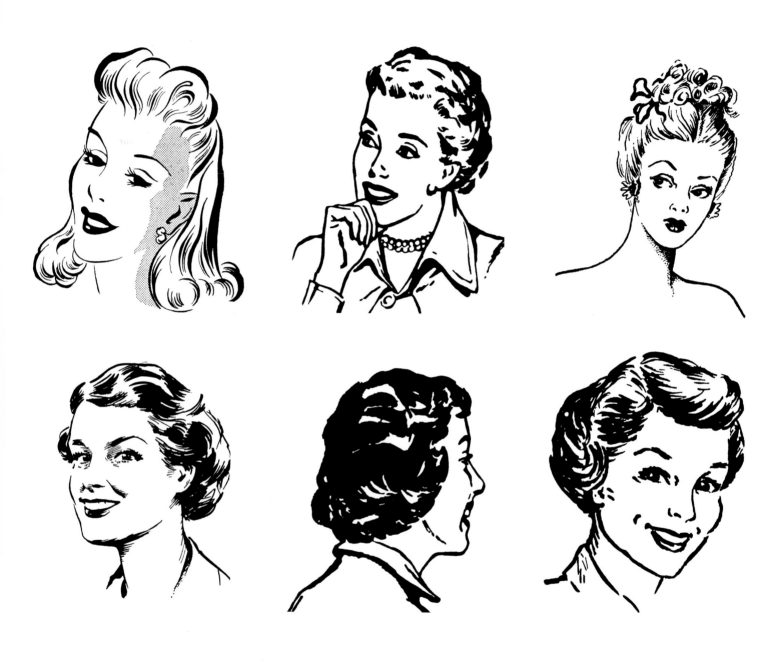

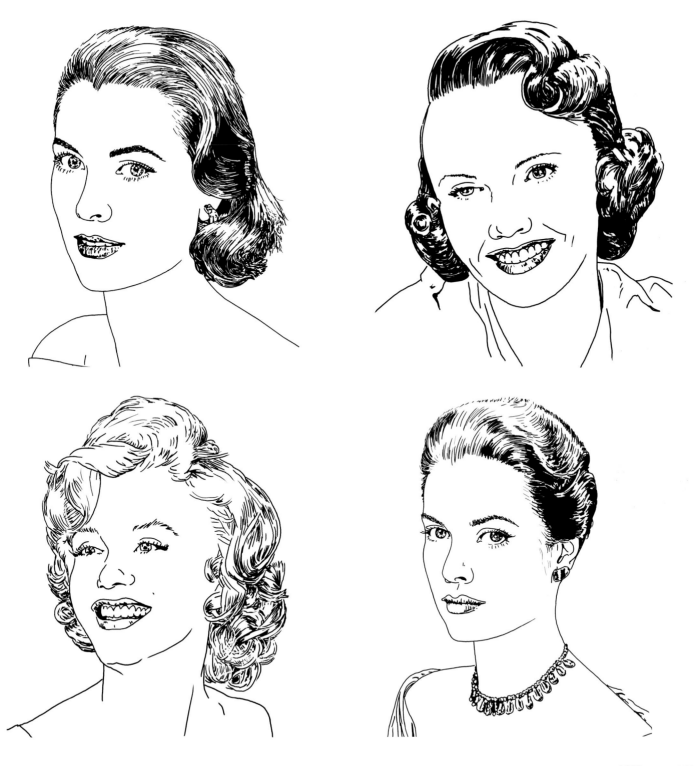

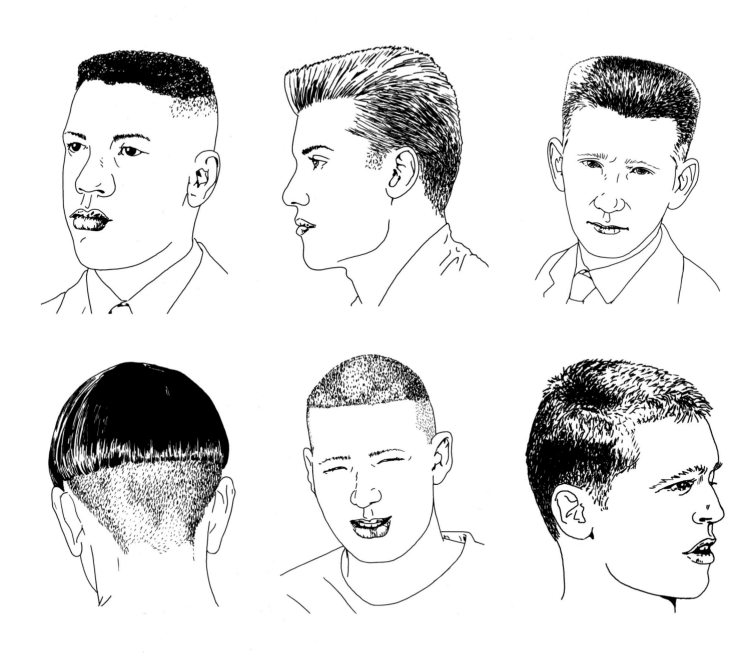

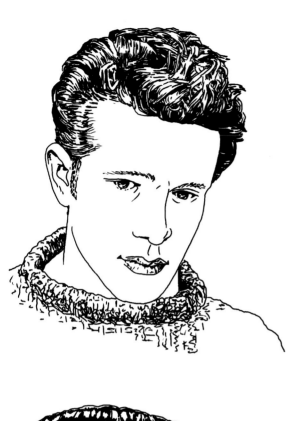

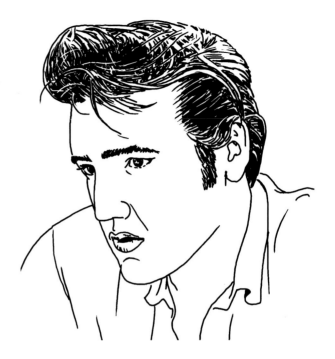

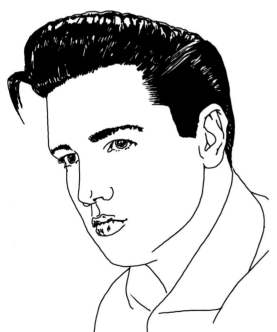

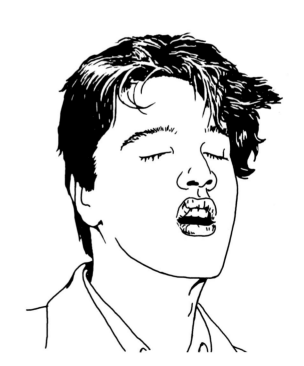

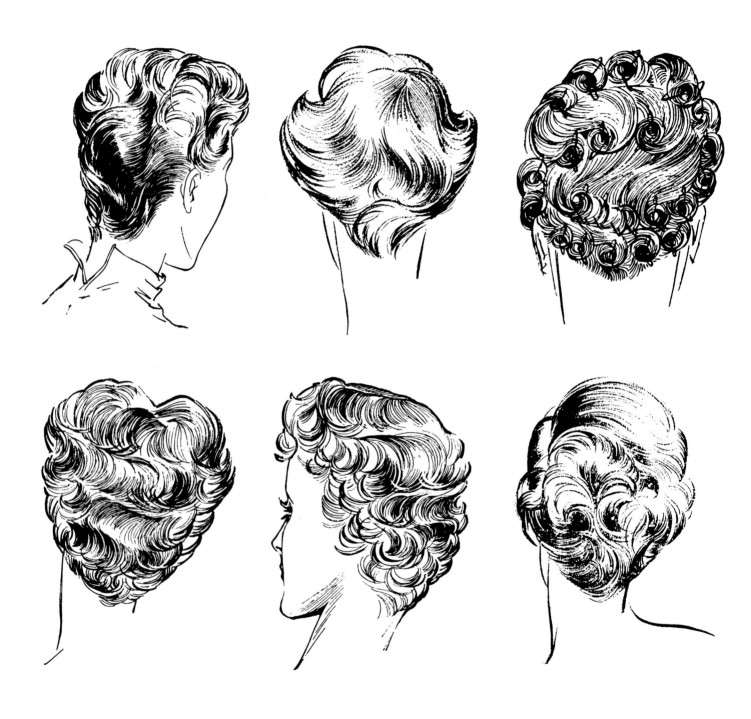

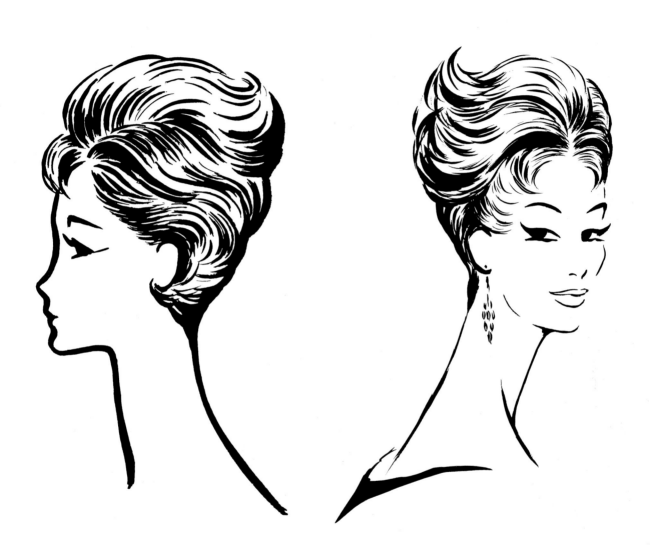

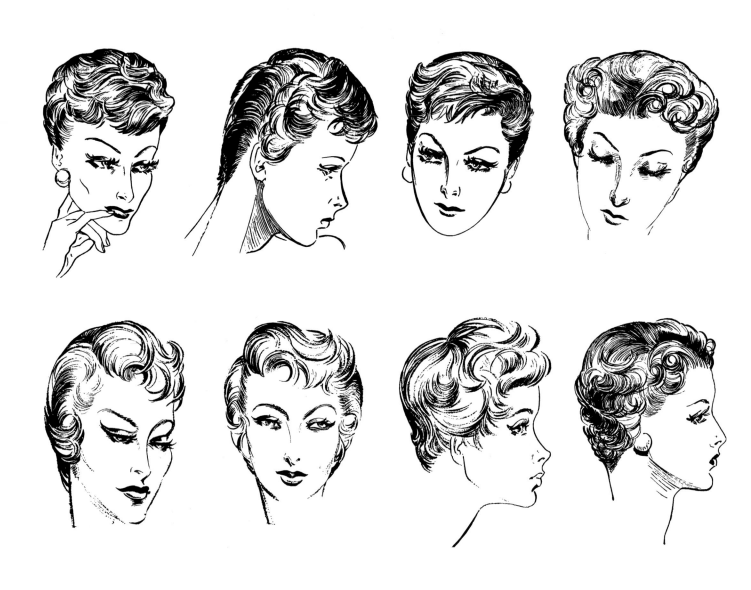

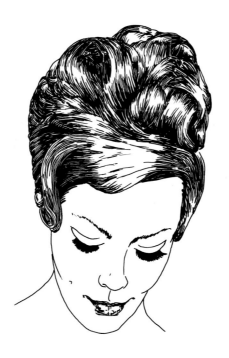

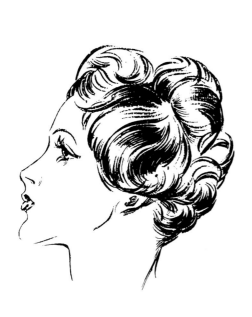

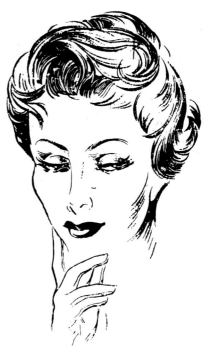

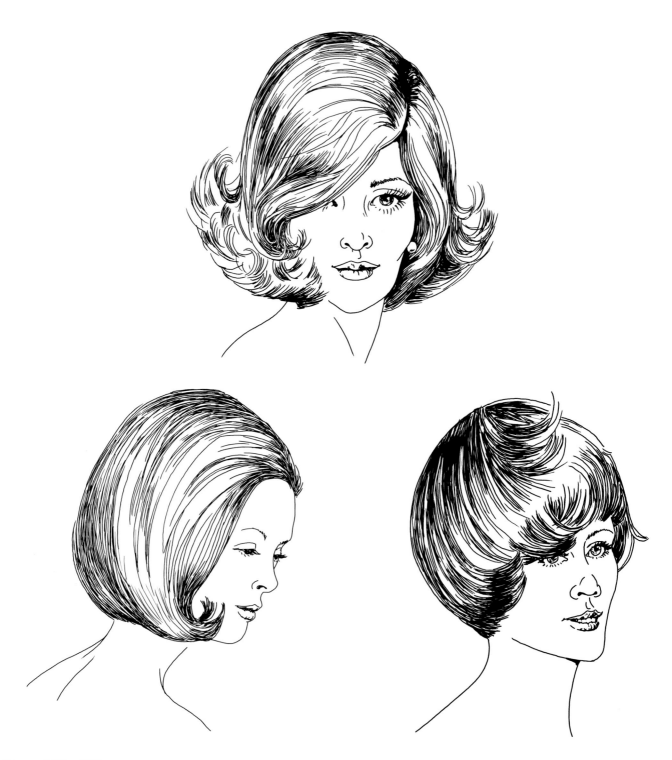

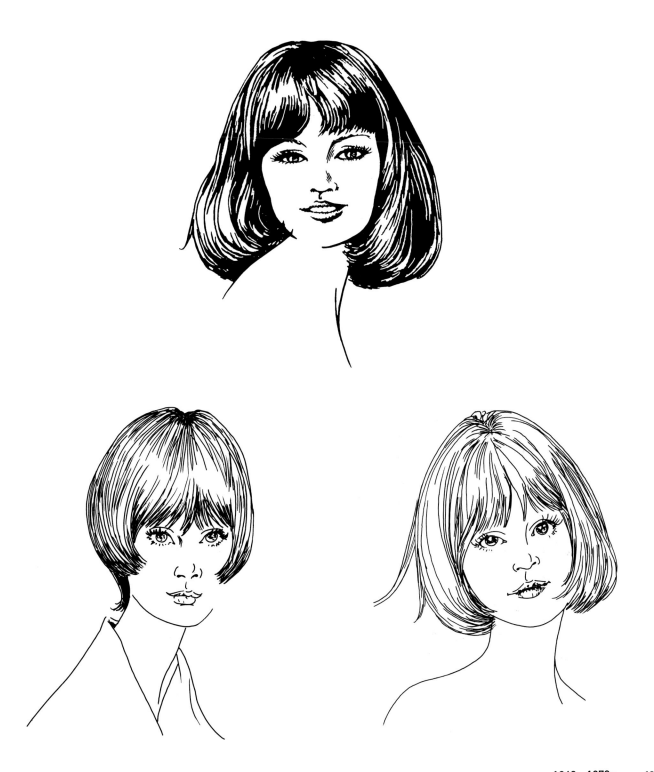

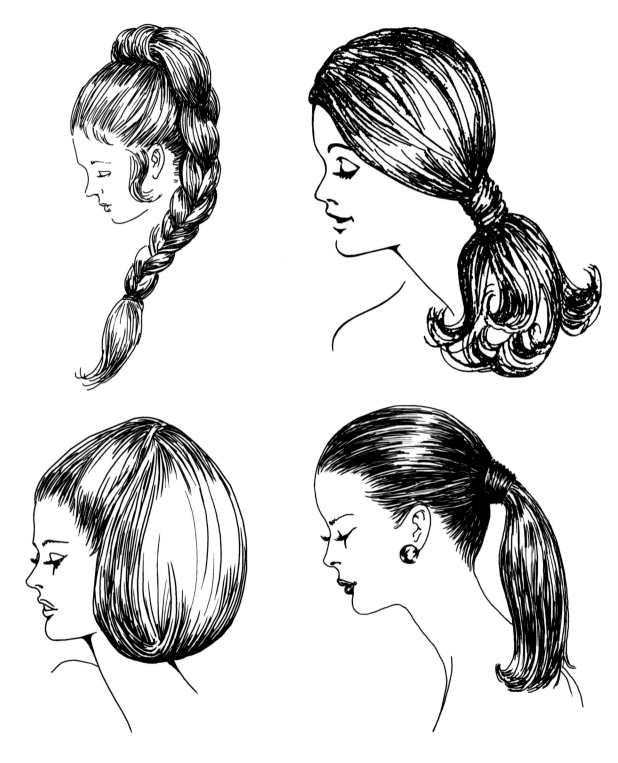

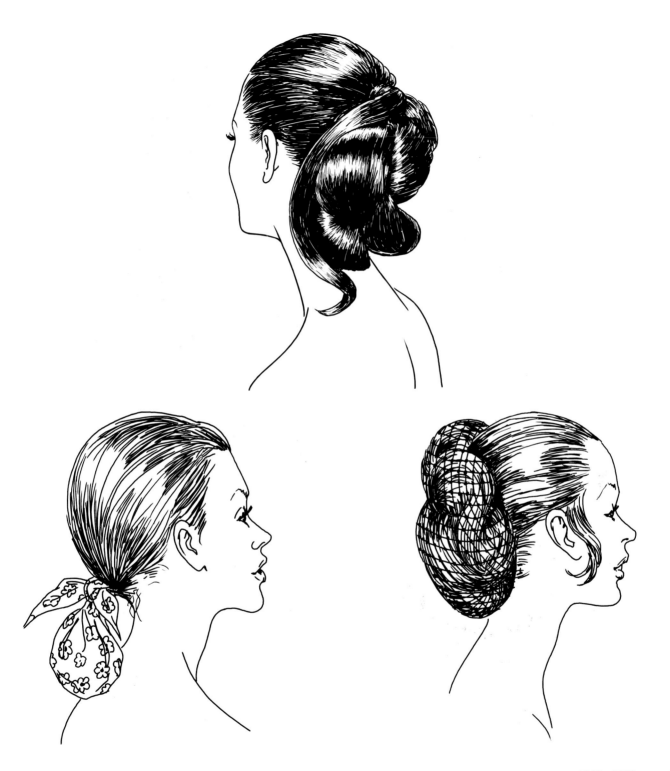

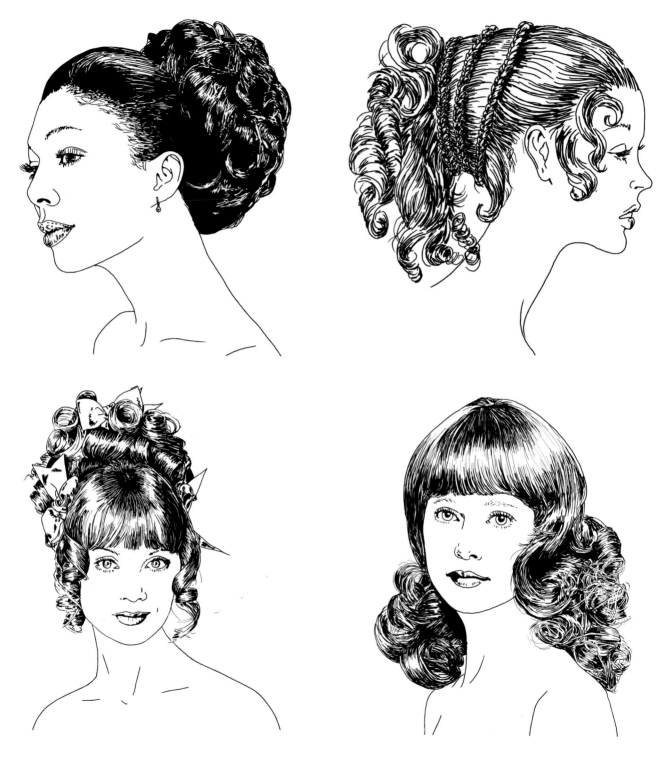

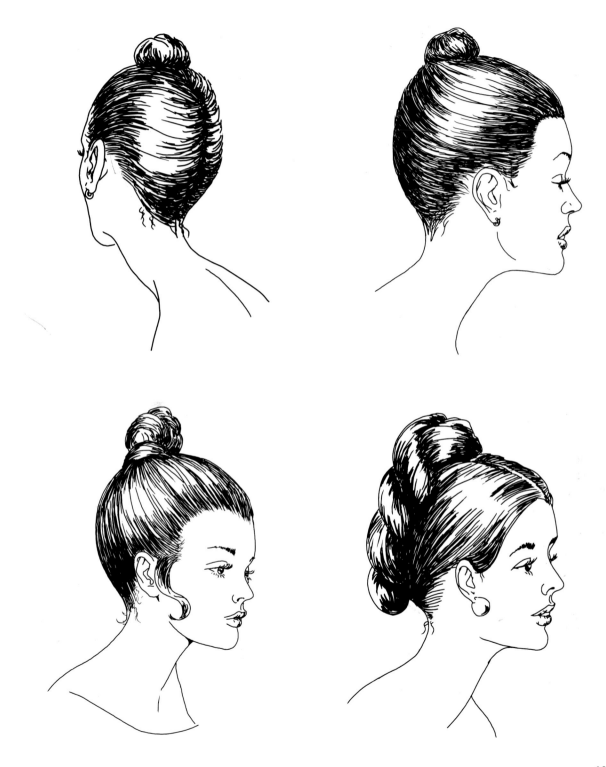

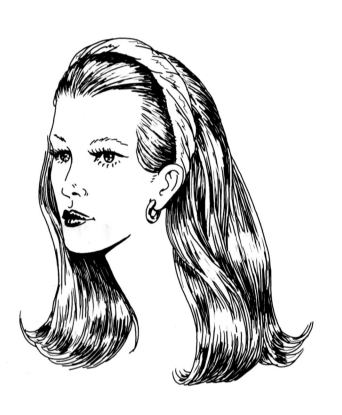
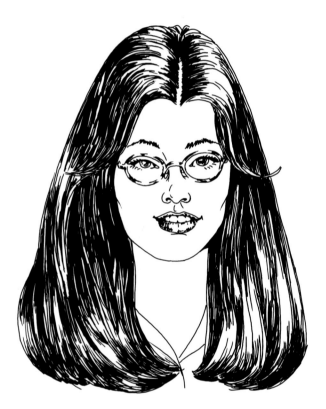

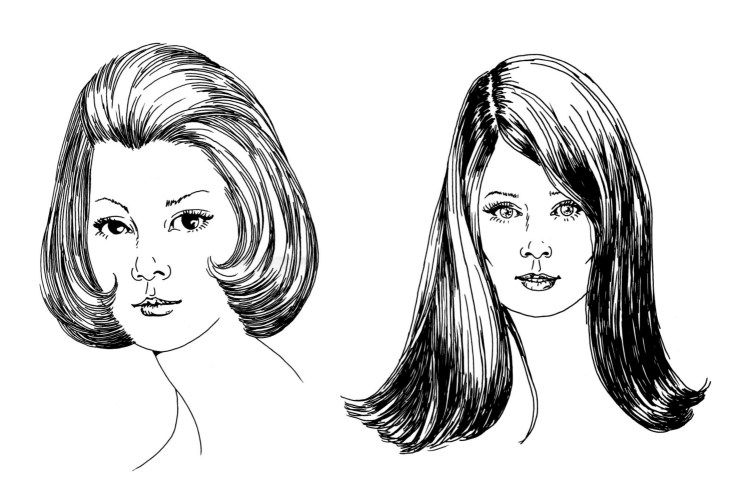

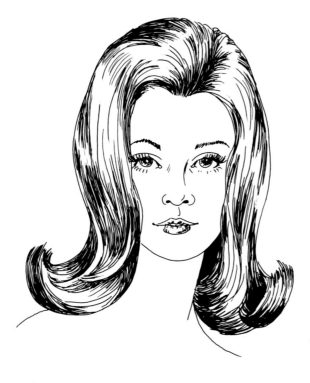

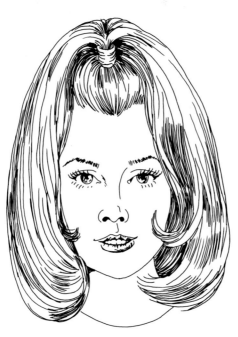

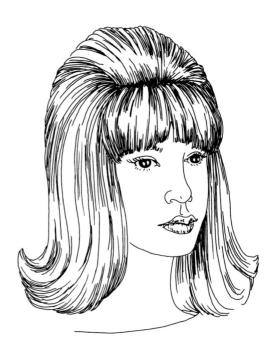

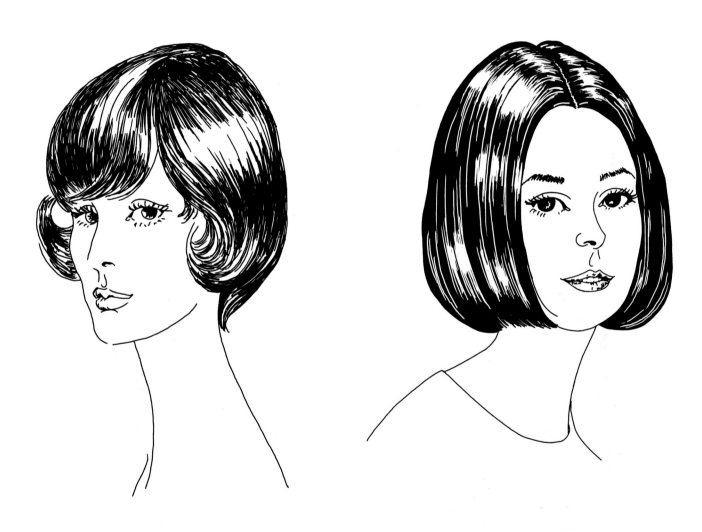

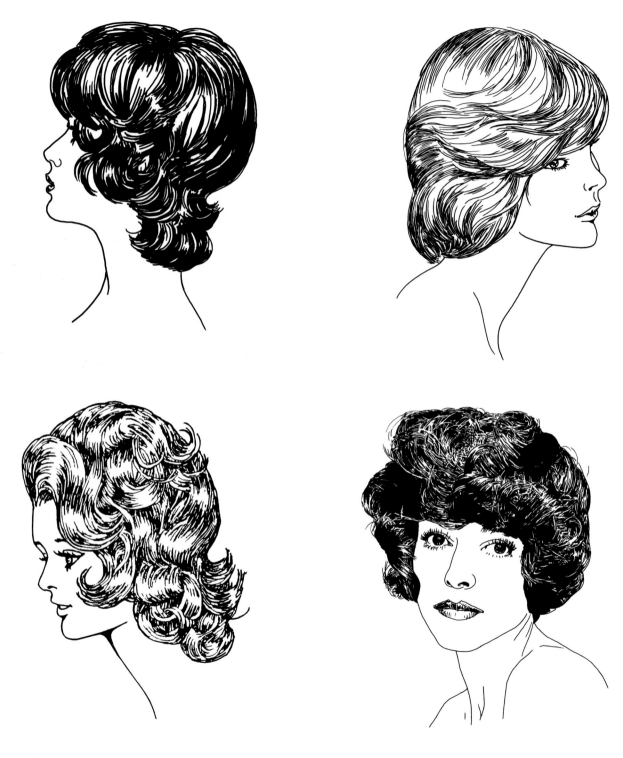

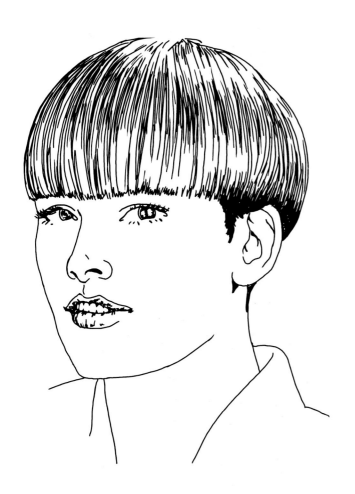
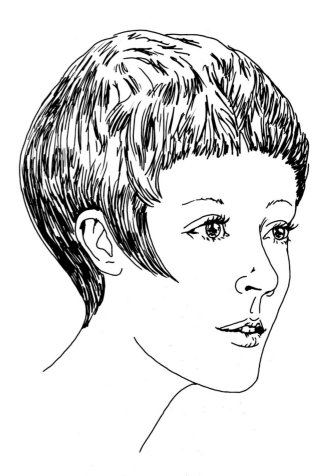

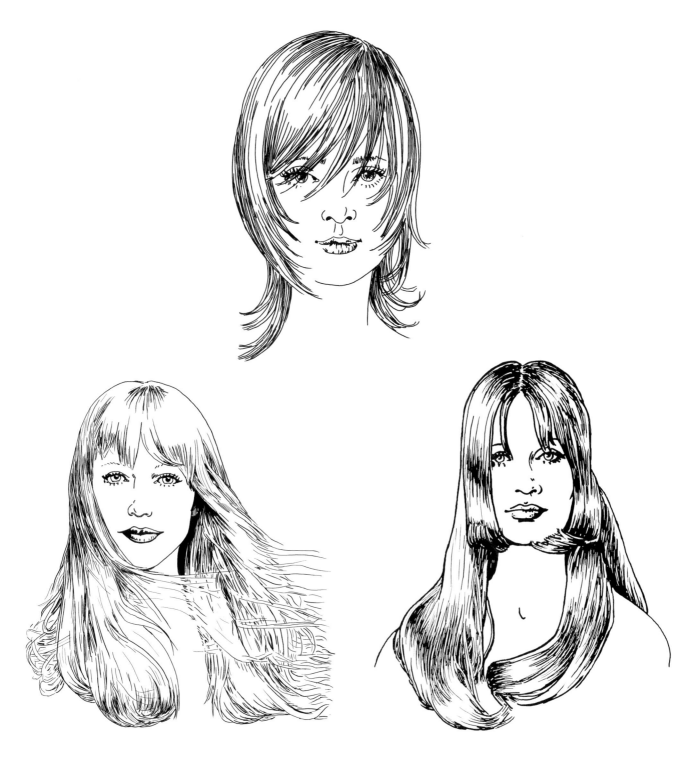

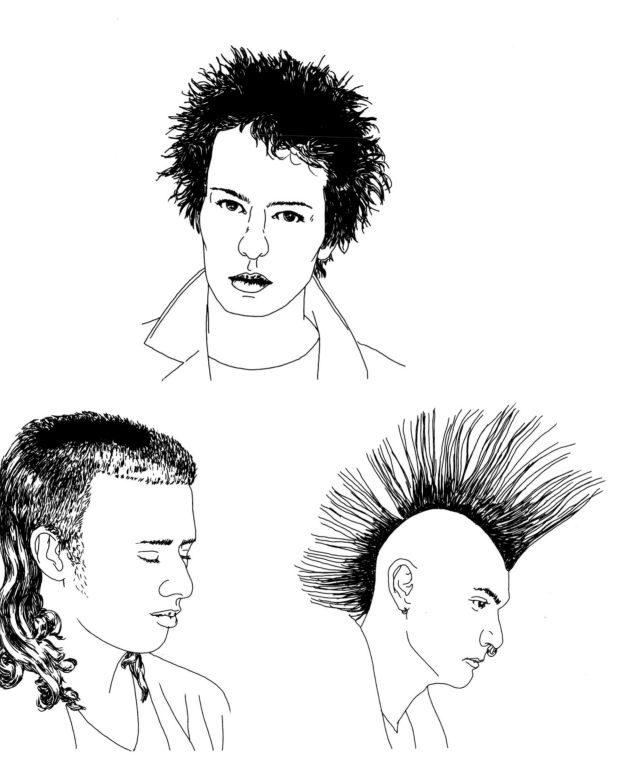

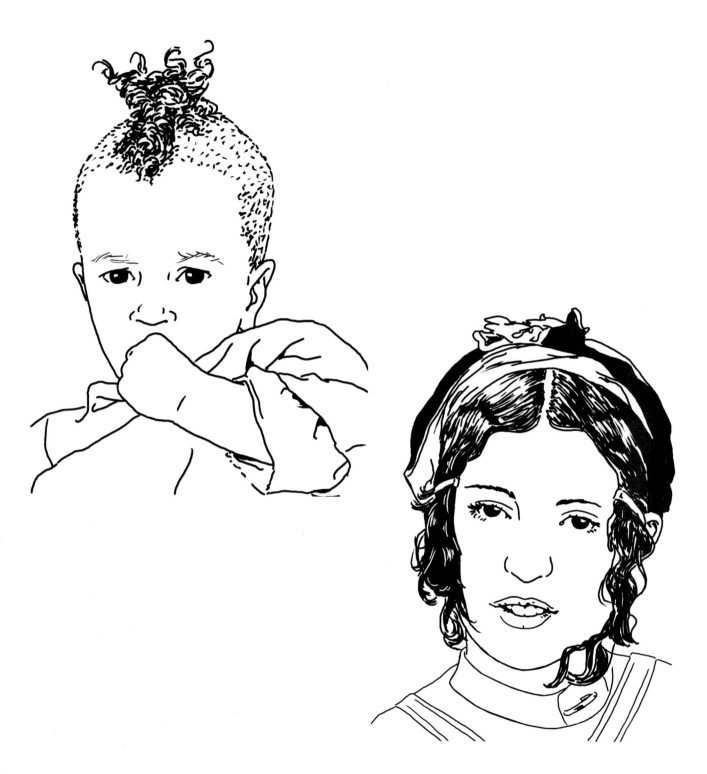

150   Morocco, Berbers

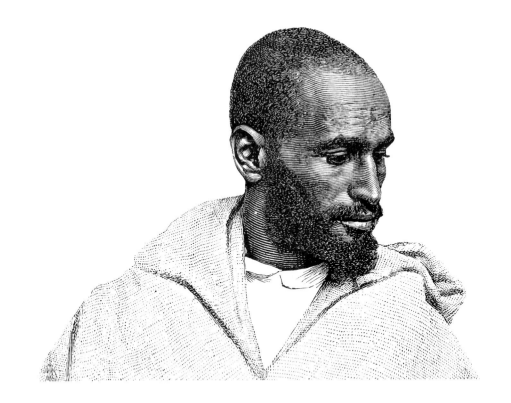

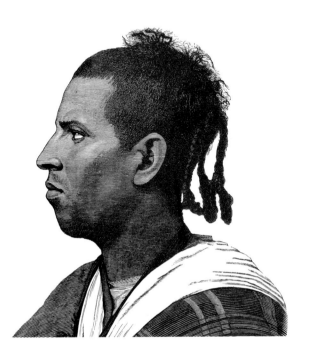

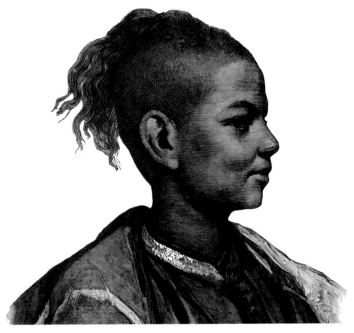

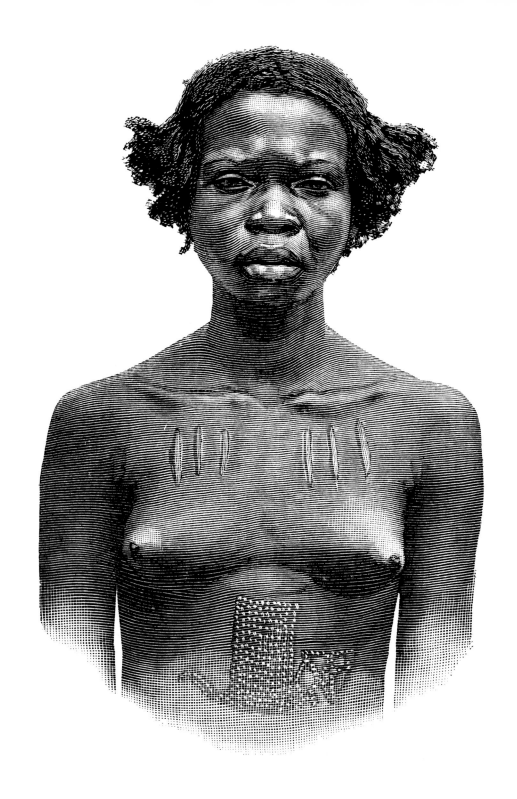

152   Sudan

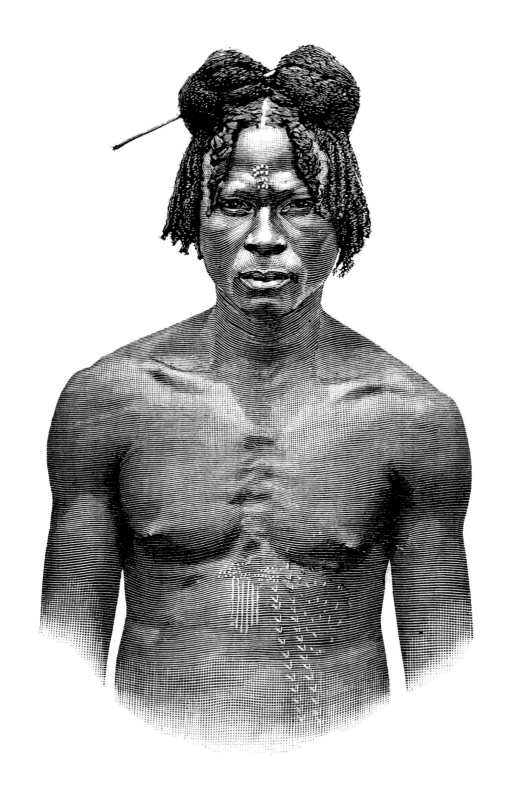

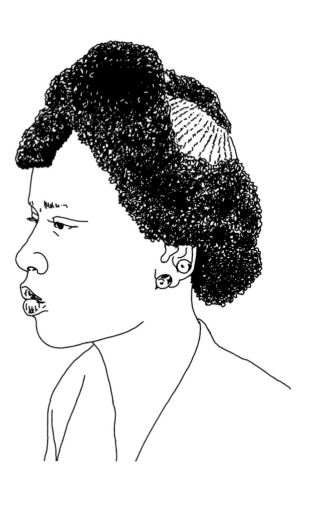
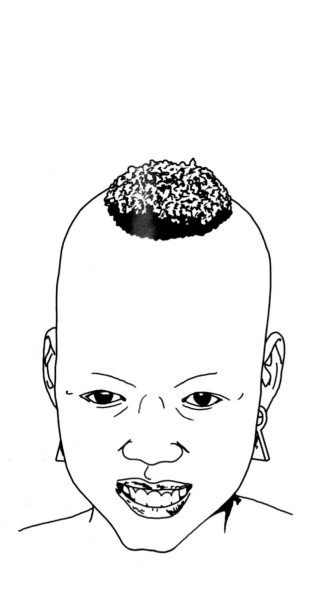

154   Sudan

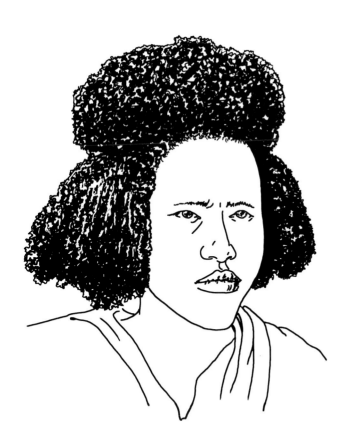
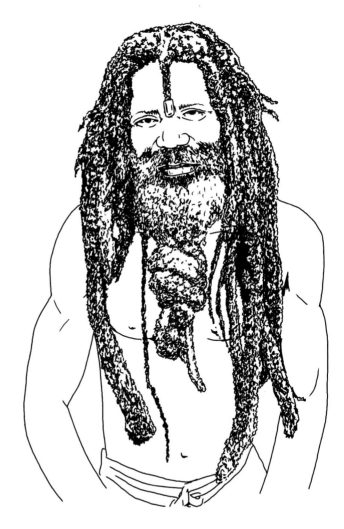

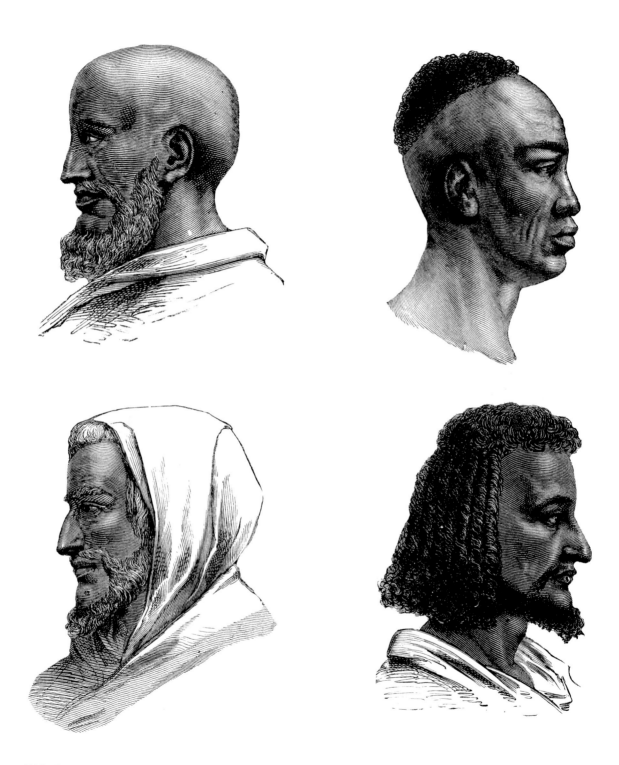

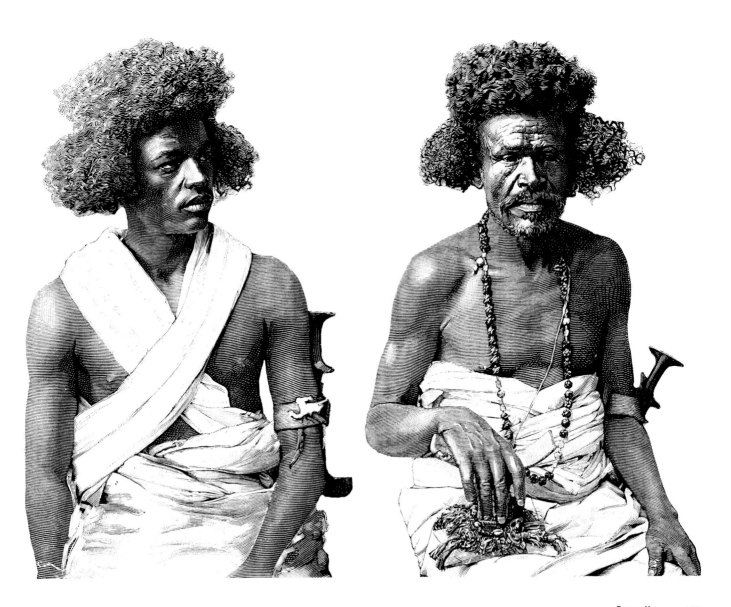

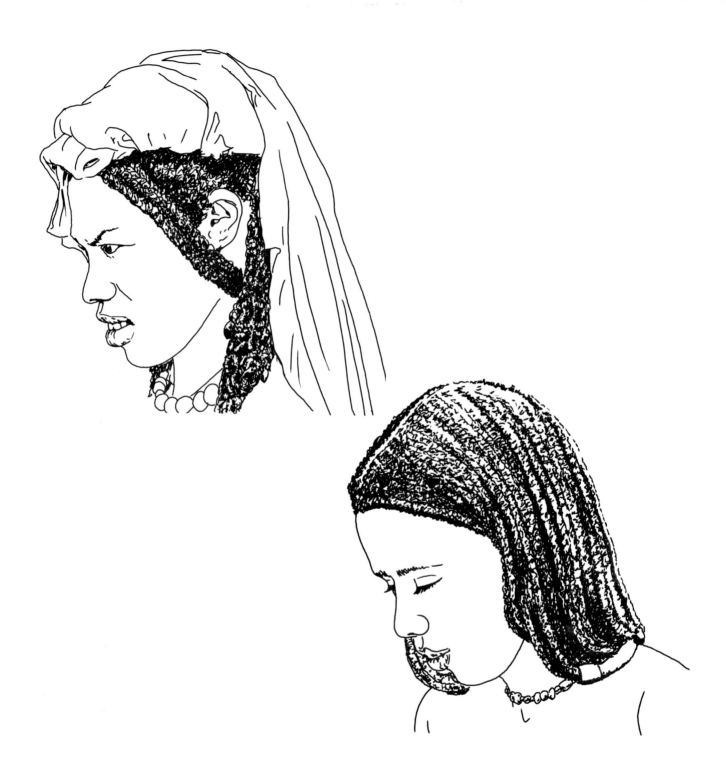

158   Somalia

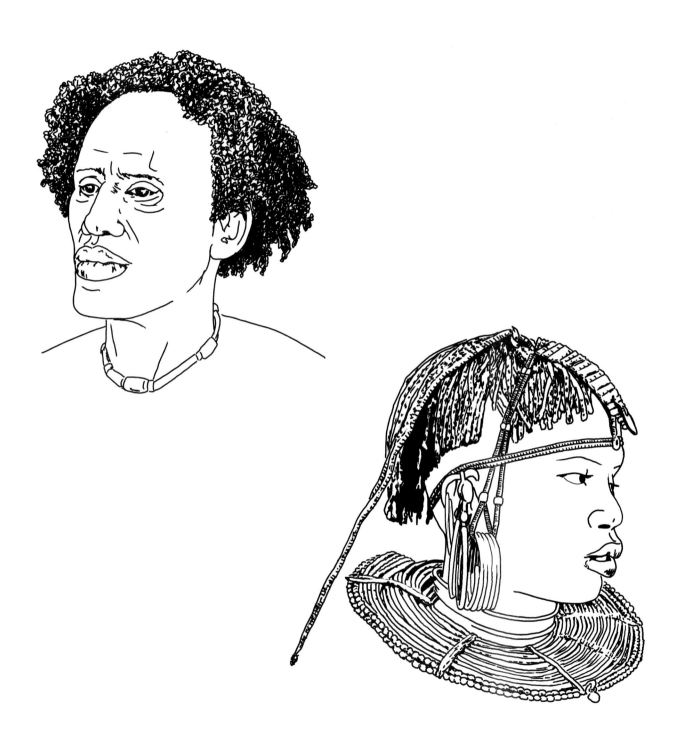

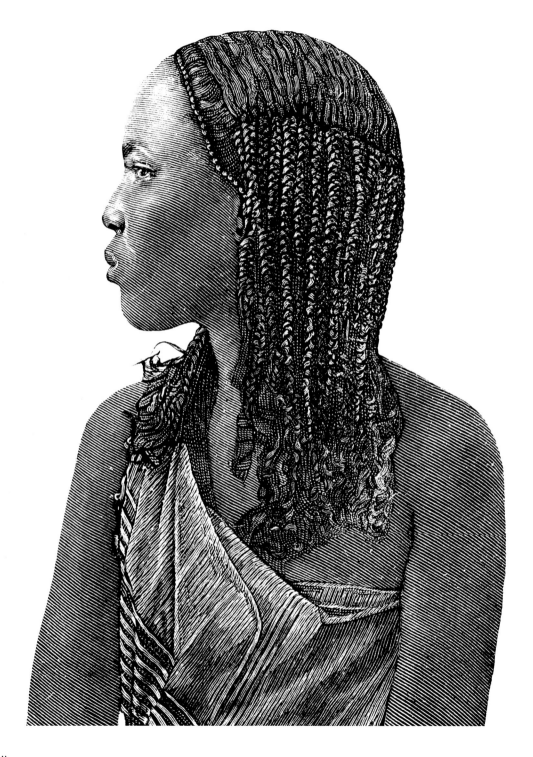

160   Somalia

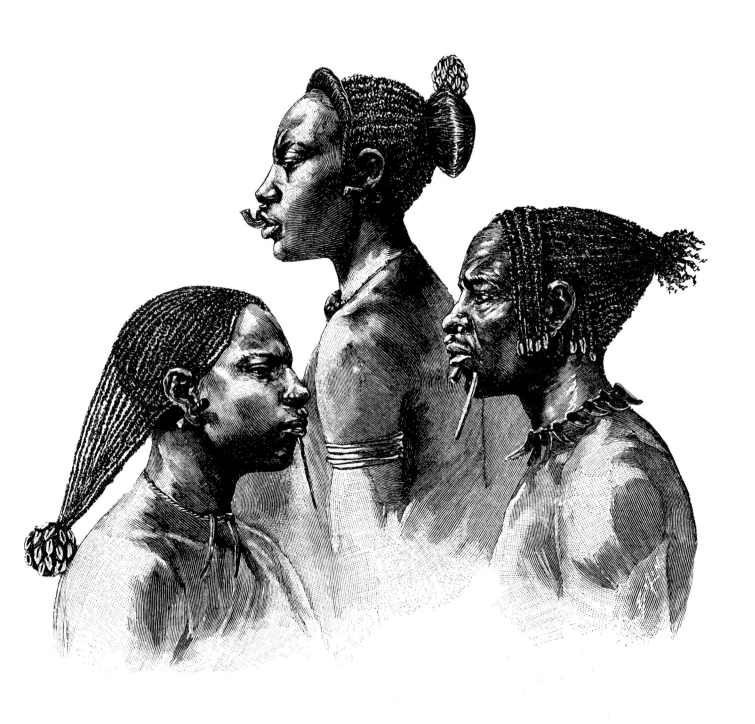

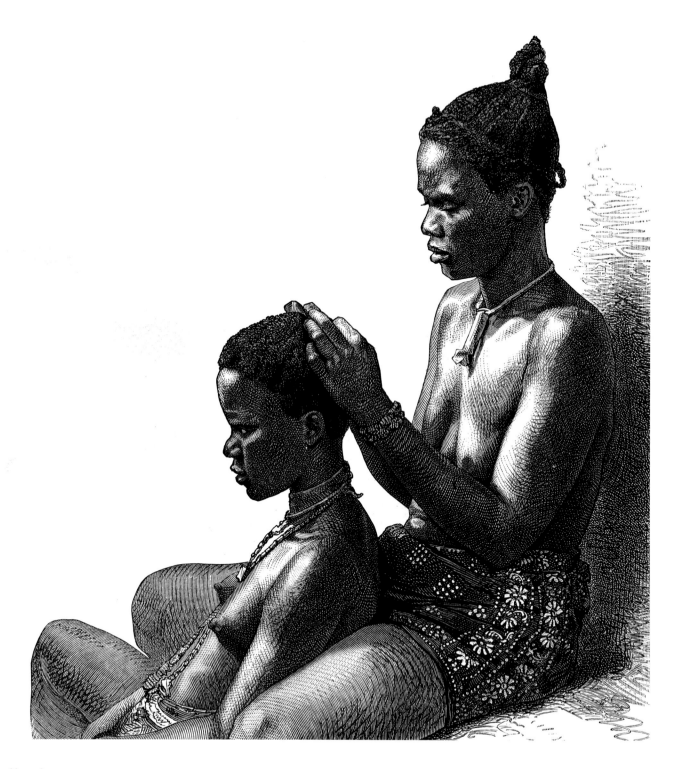

162   Uganda

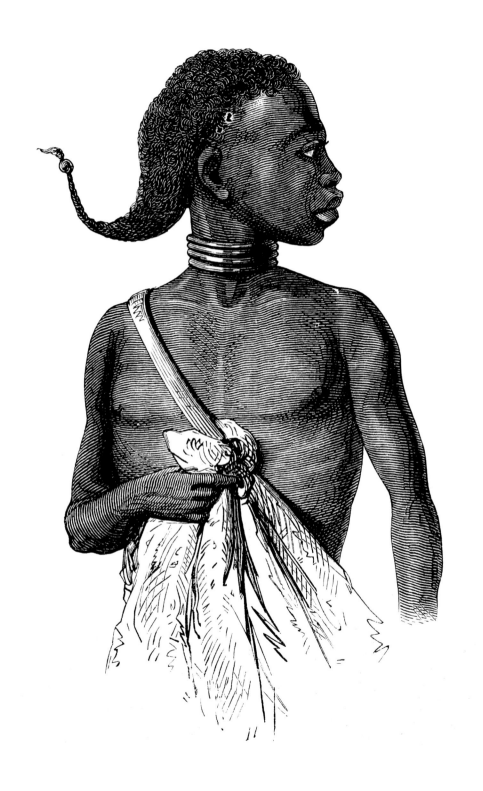

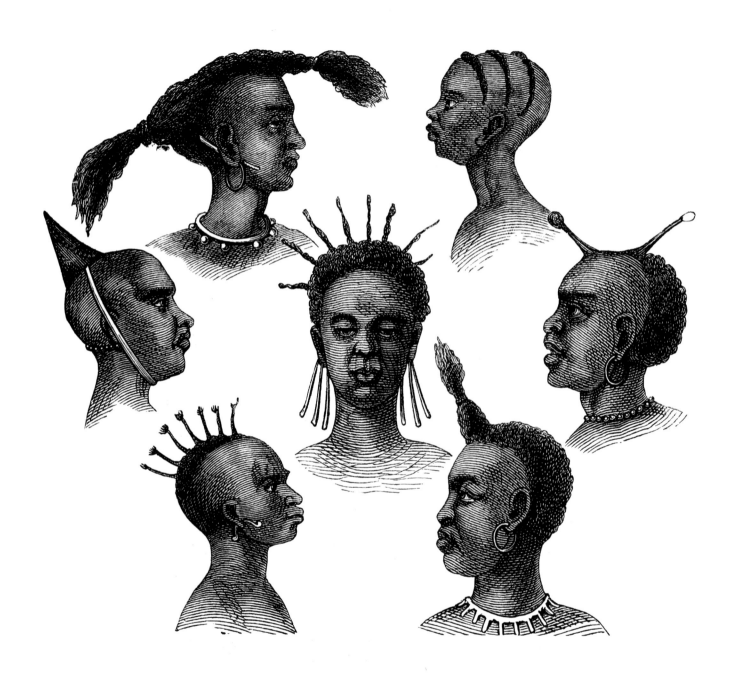

164   Tanzania

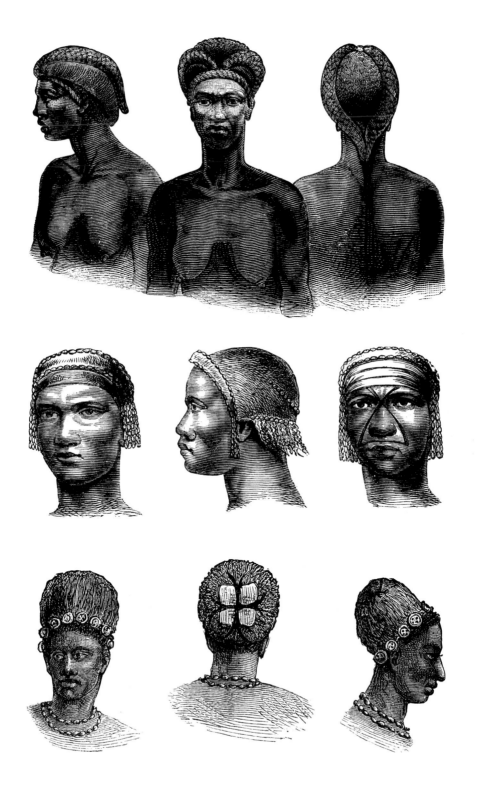

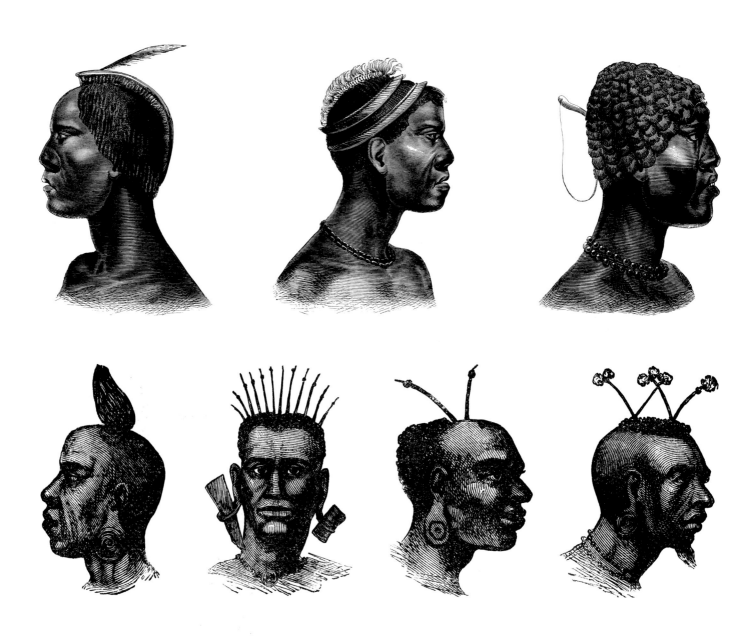

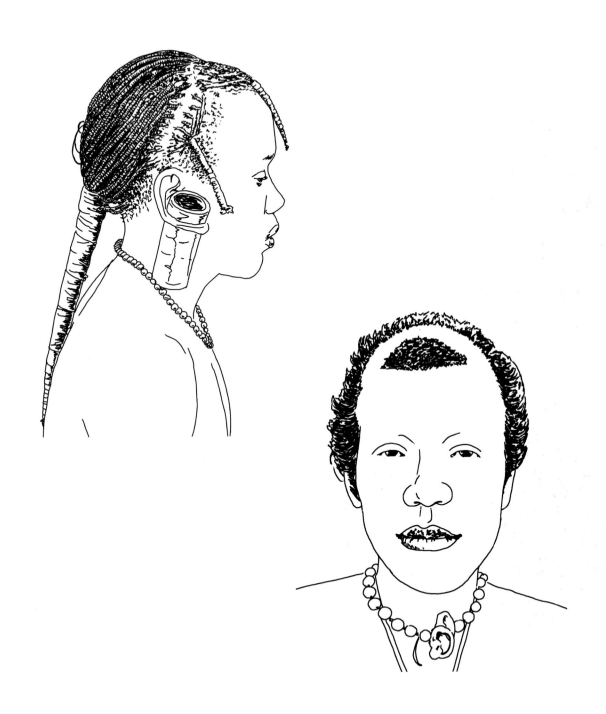

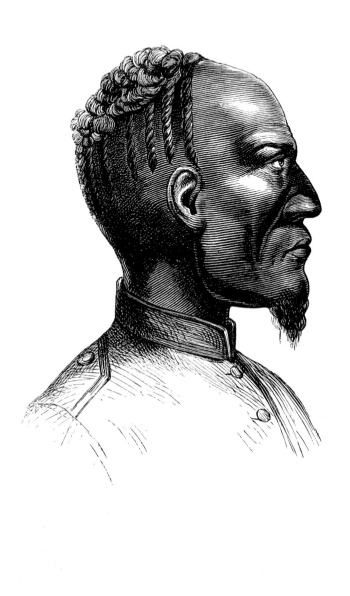
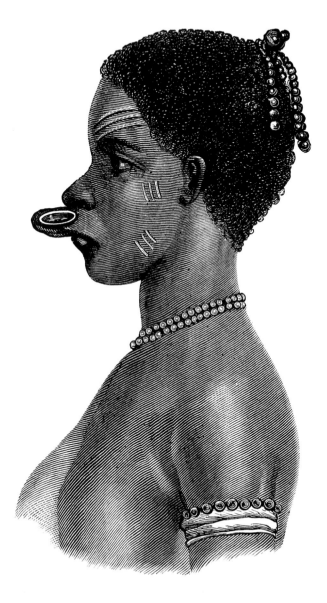

168   Zambia

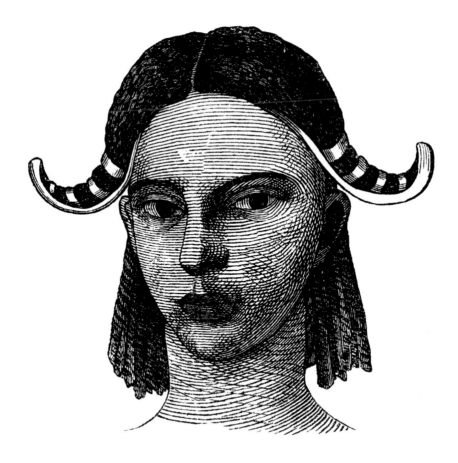

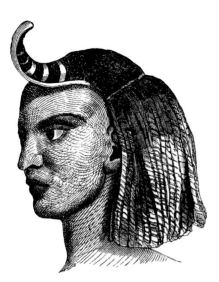

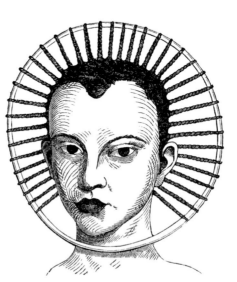

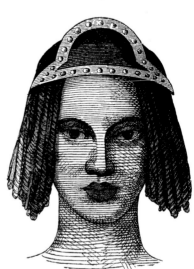

Zambia/Mozambique   169

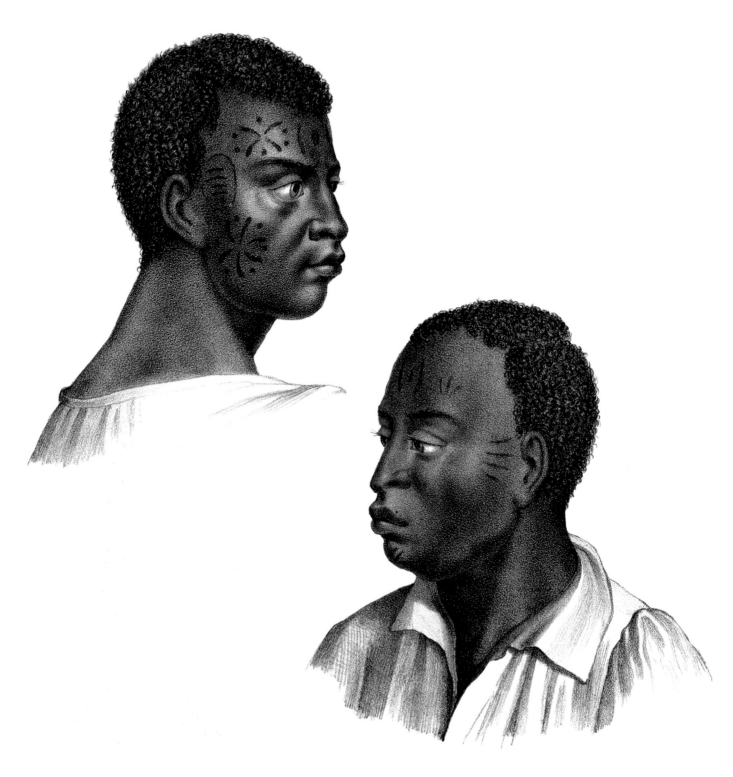

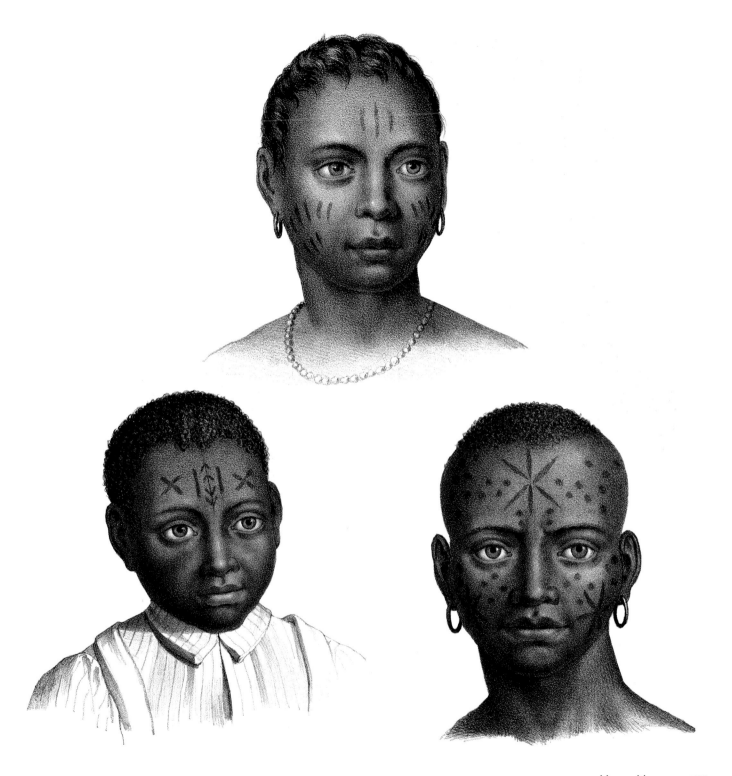

Mozambique 171

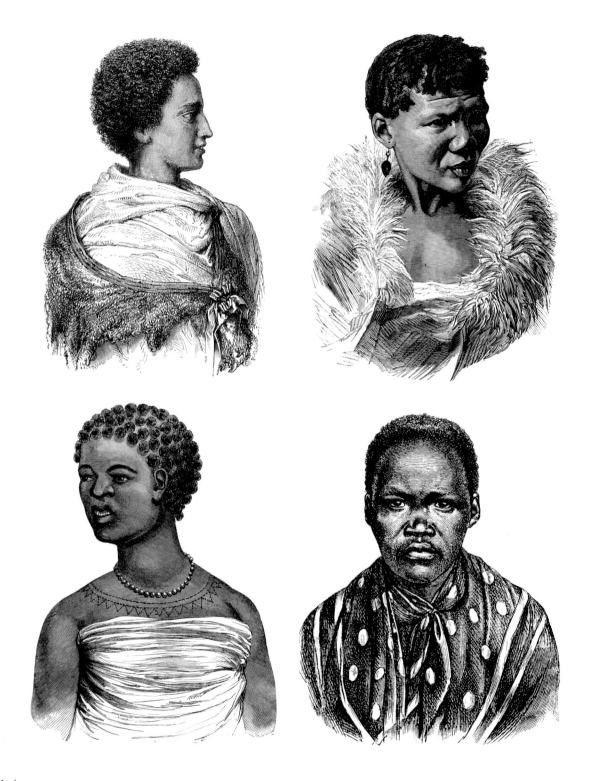

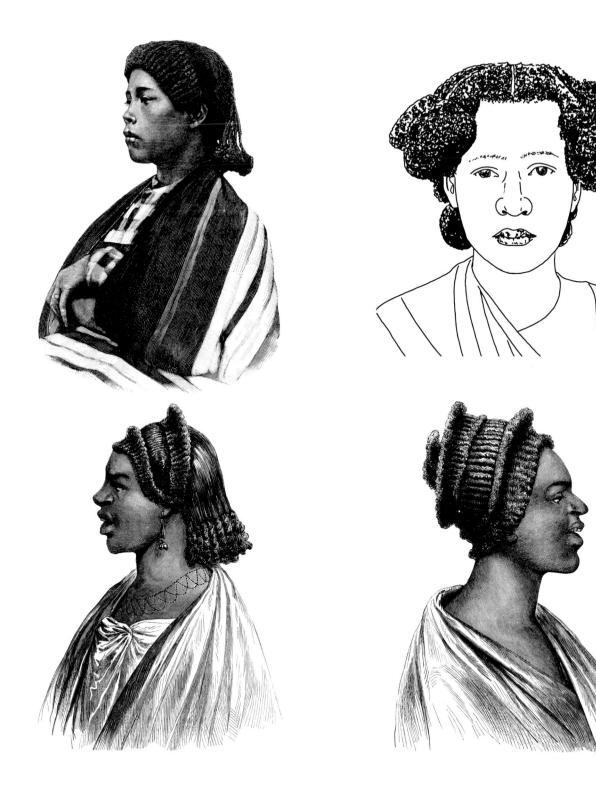

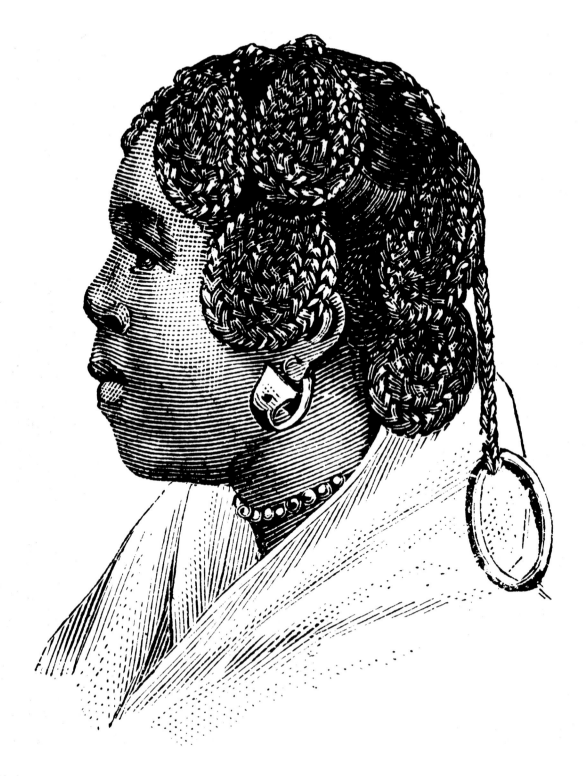

174   Madagascar

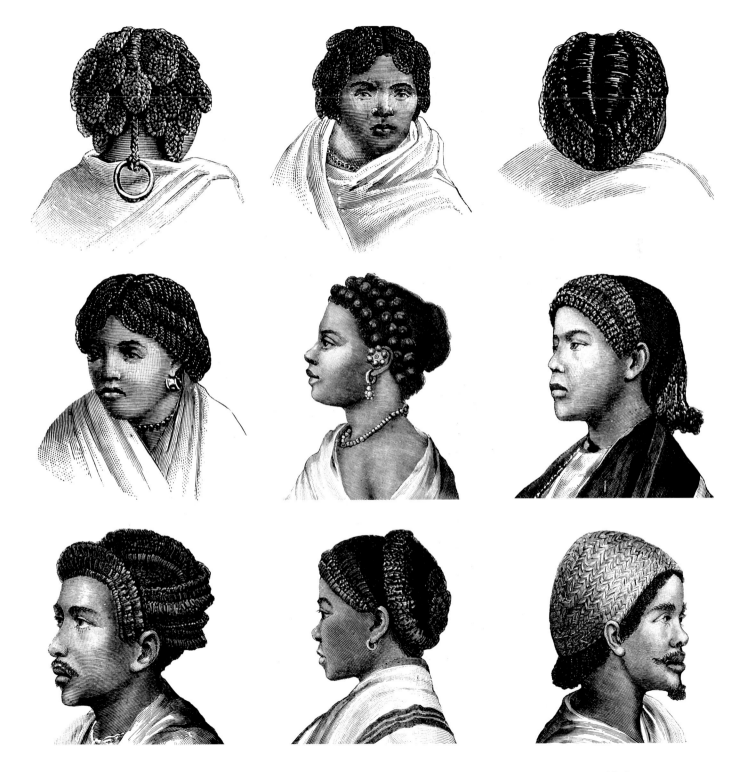

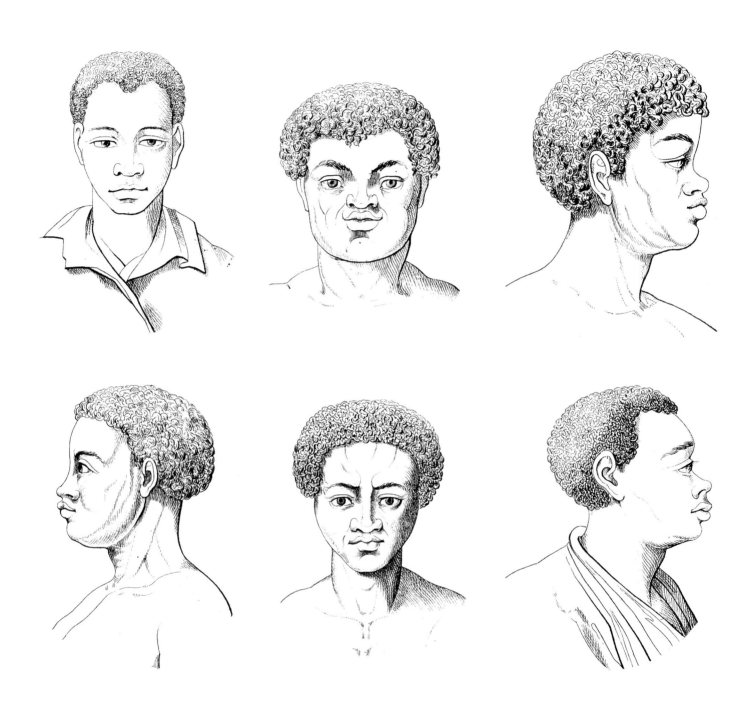

176   South Africa, Bushmen

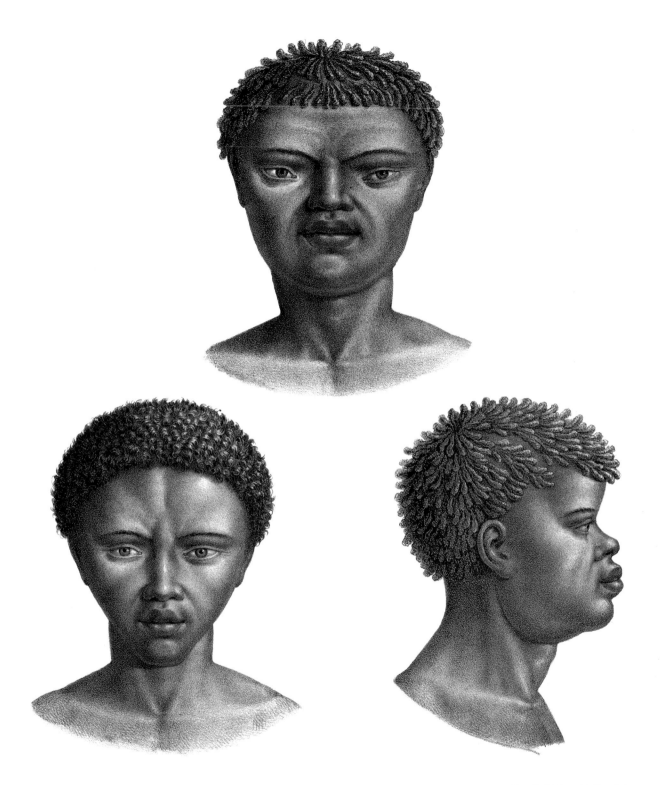

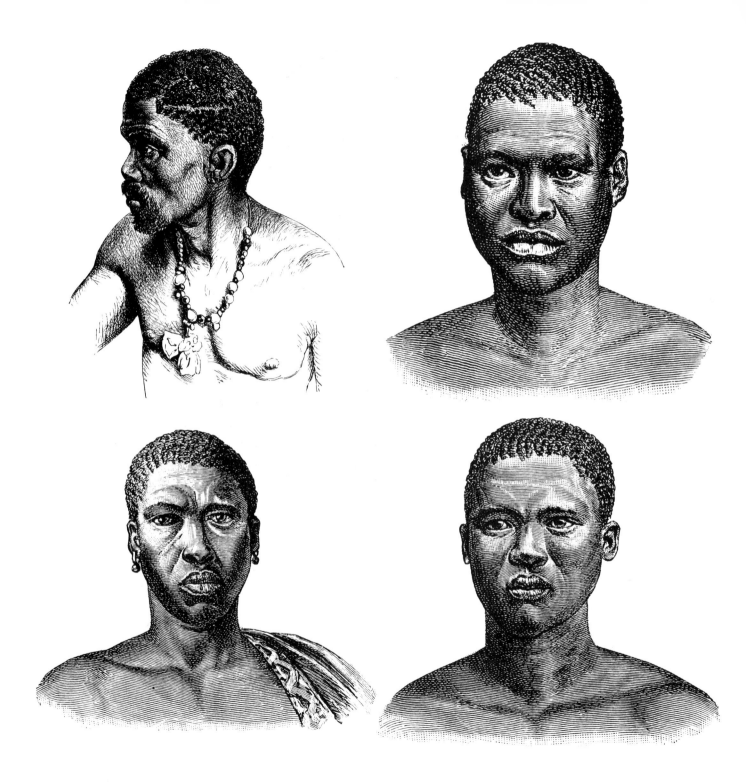

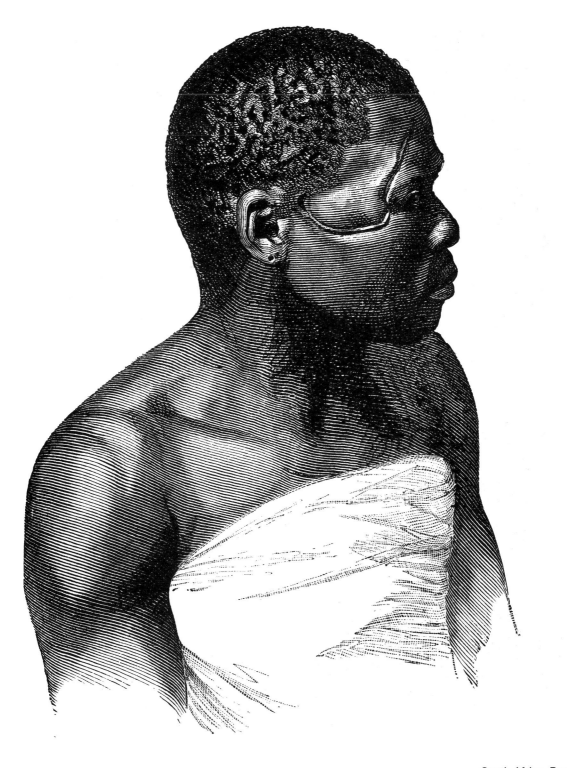

South Africa, Bantu 179

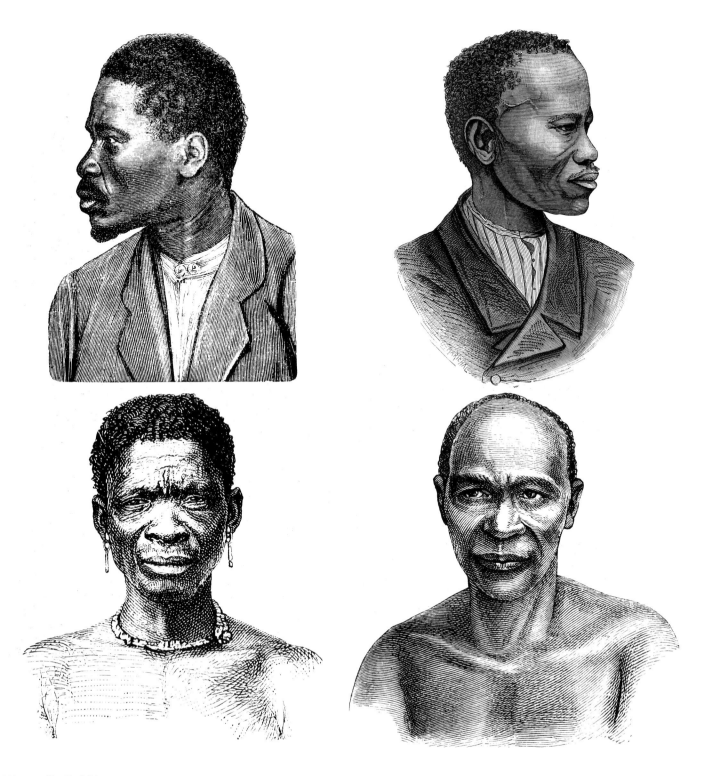

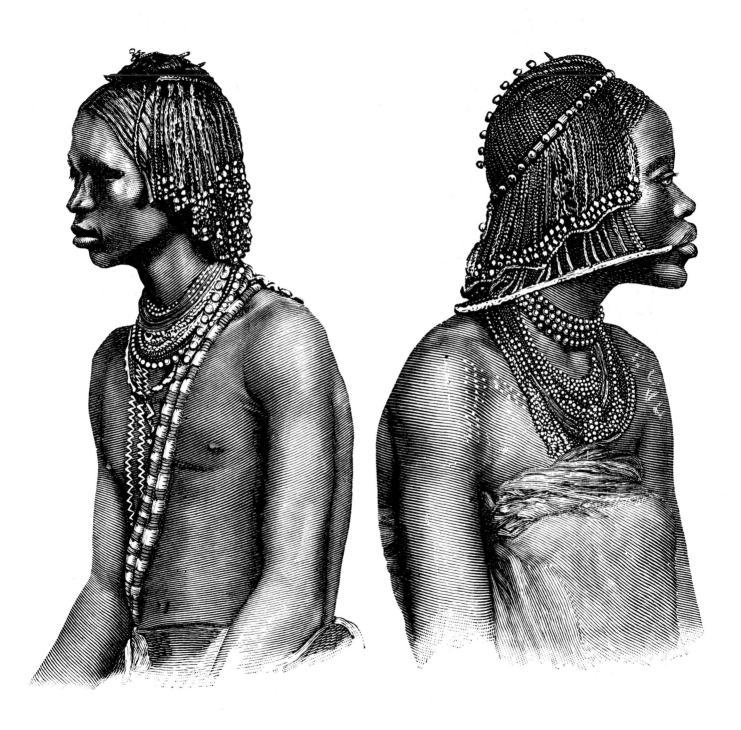

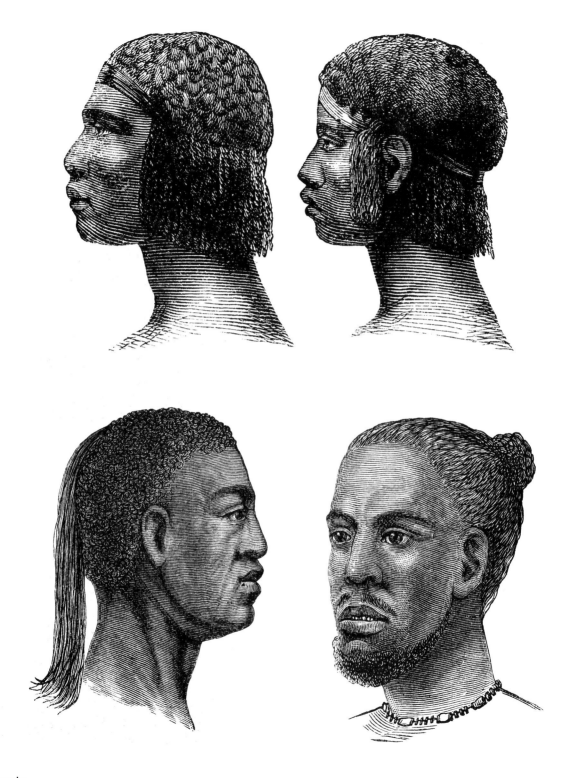

182 Angola

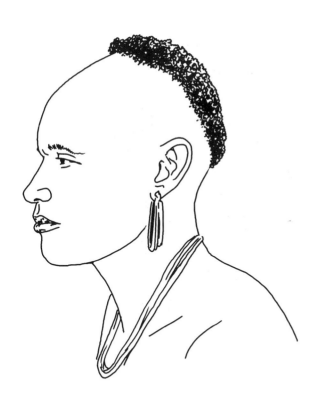

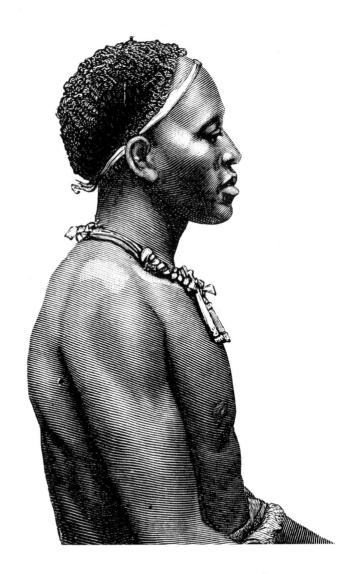

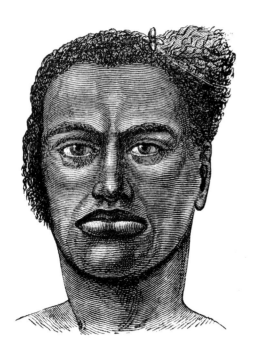
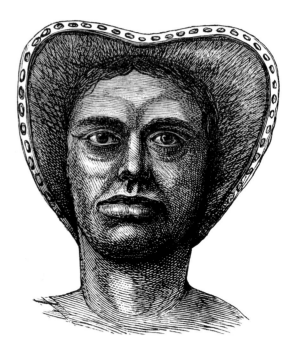
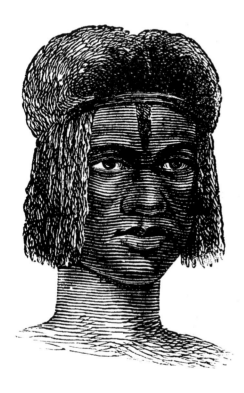
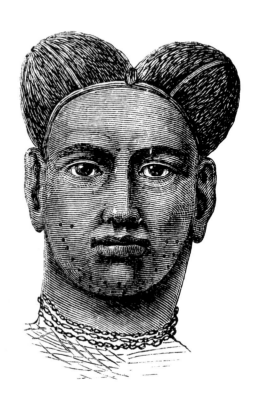

184 Congo

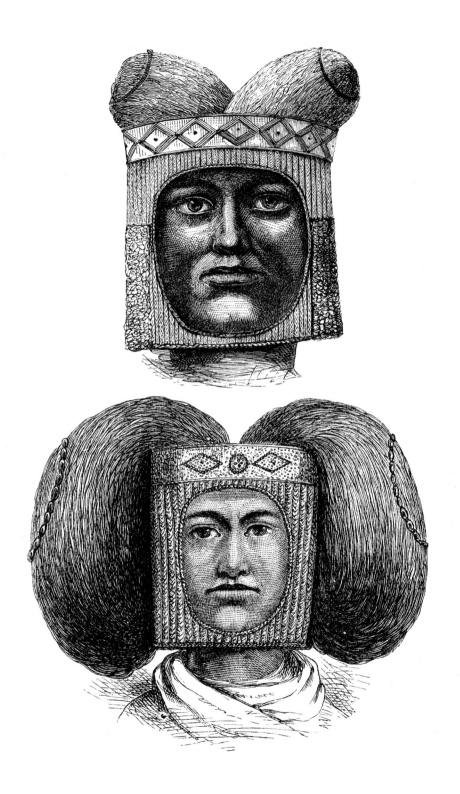

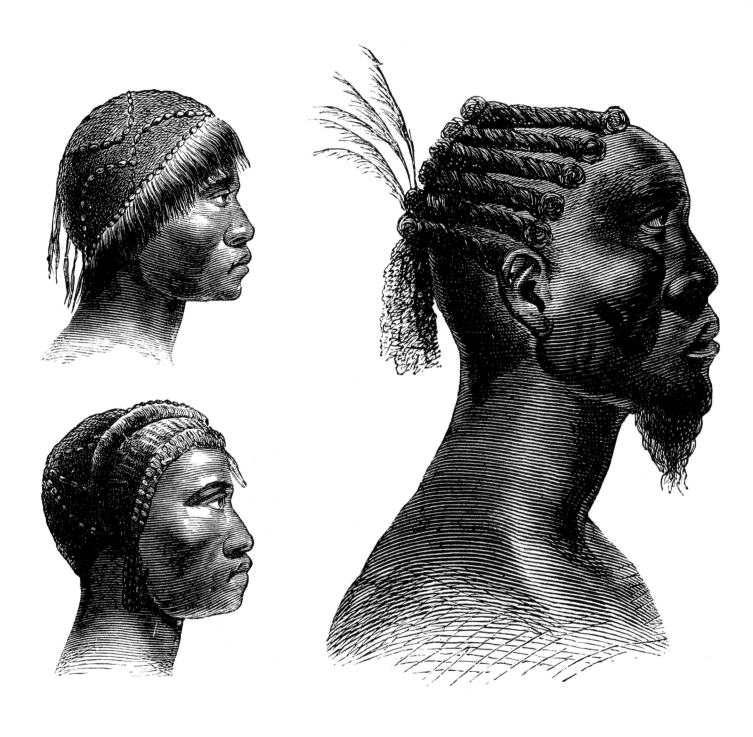

186 Congo

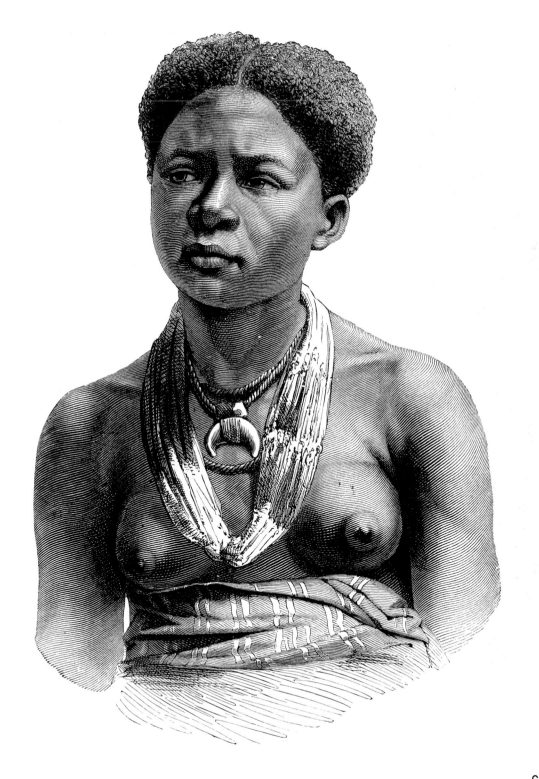

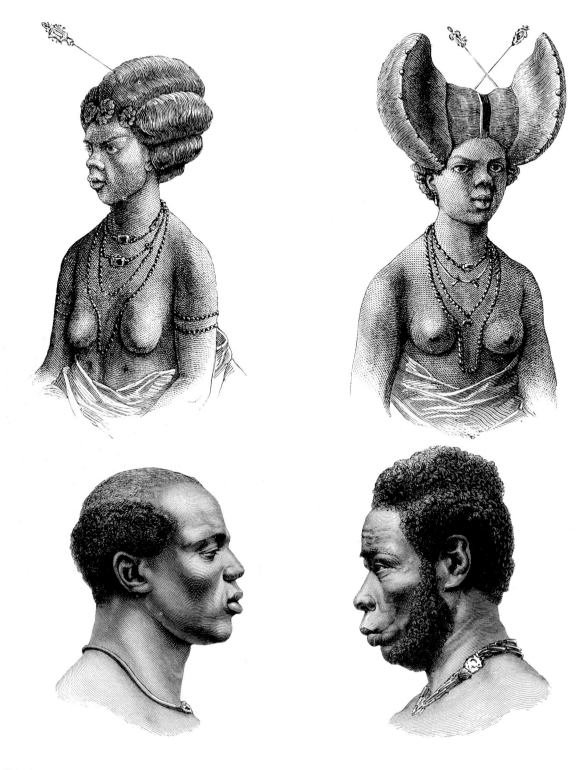

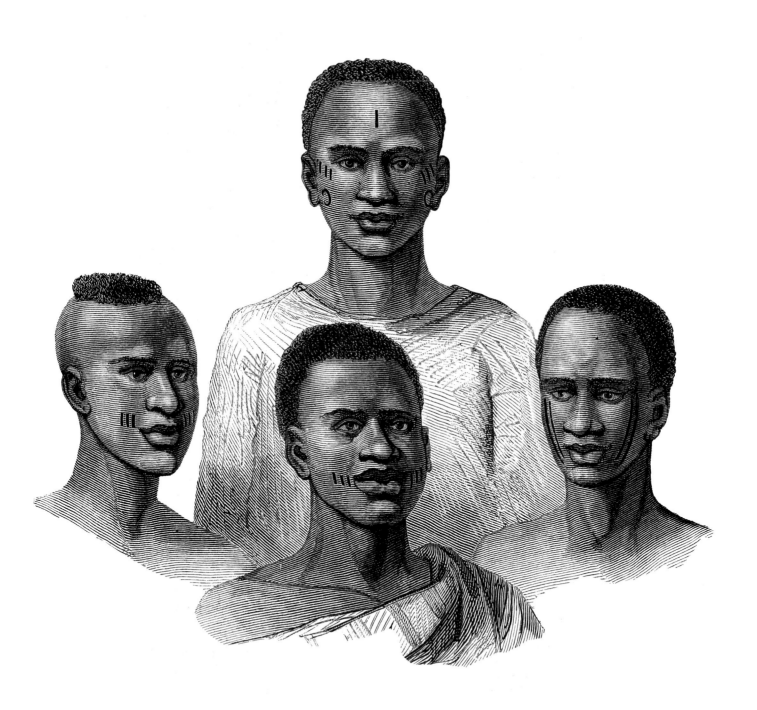

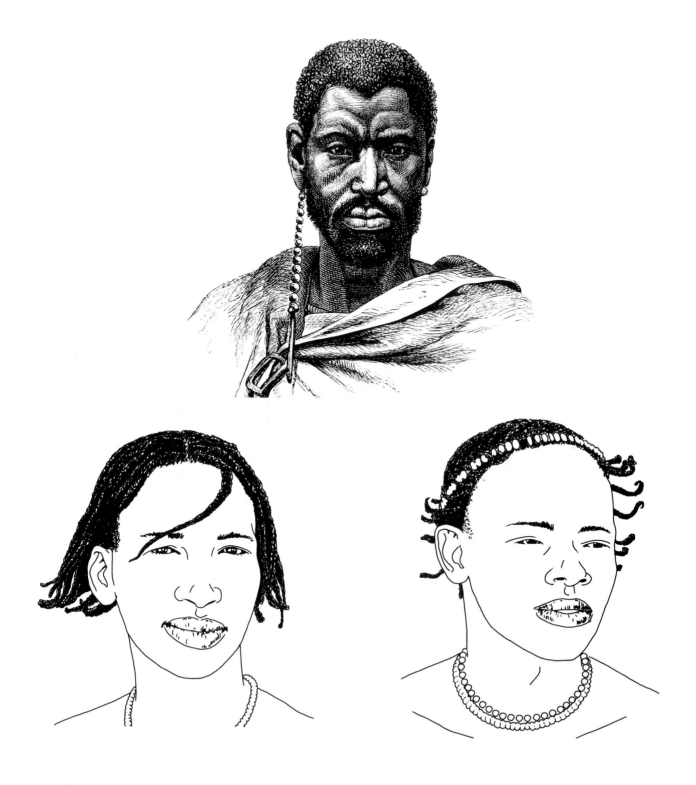

190   Chad/Niger

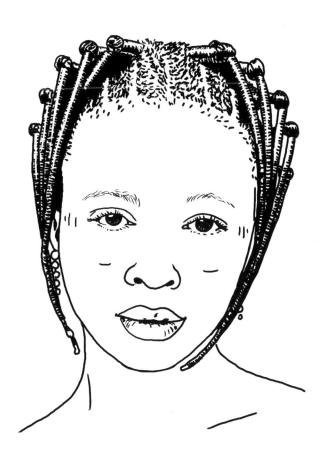

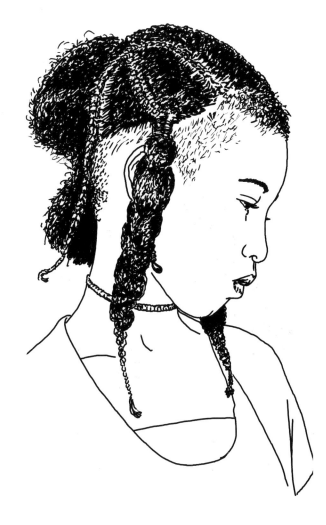

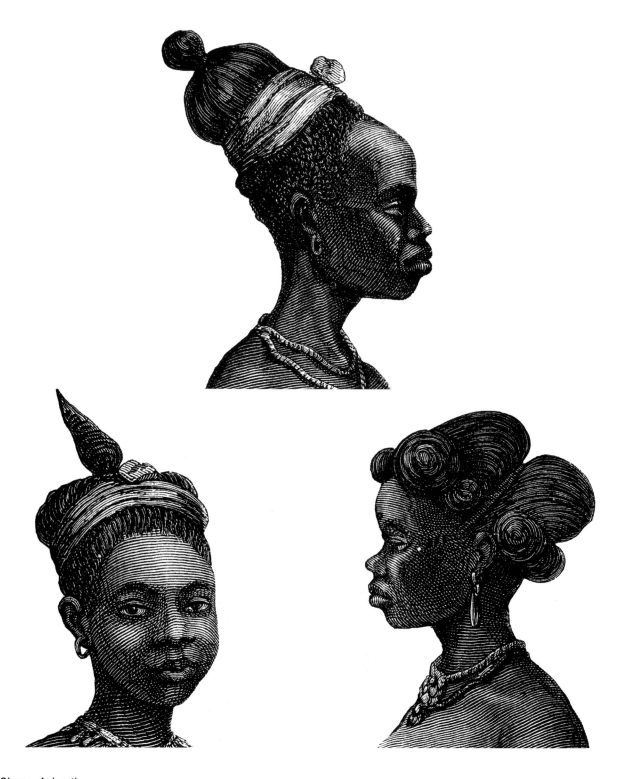

192 Ghana, Ashanti

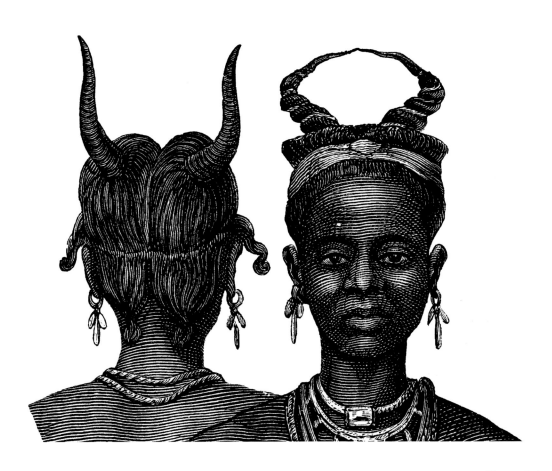

Ghana, Ashanti 193

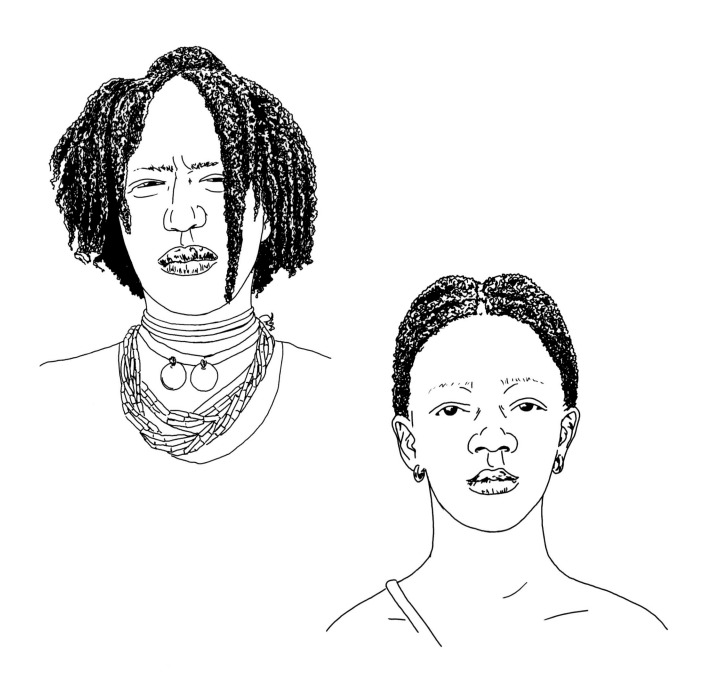

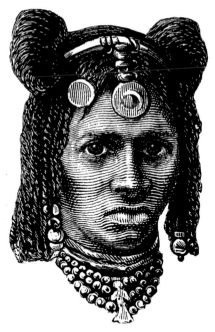

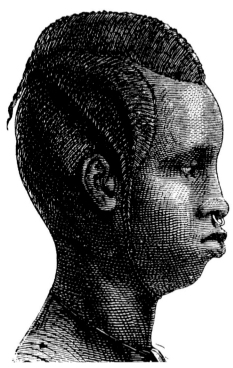

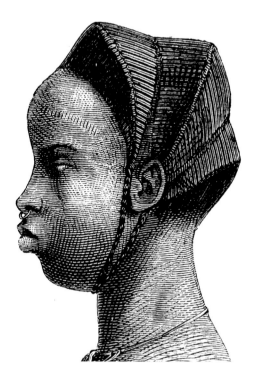

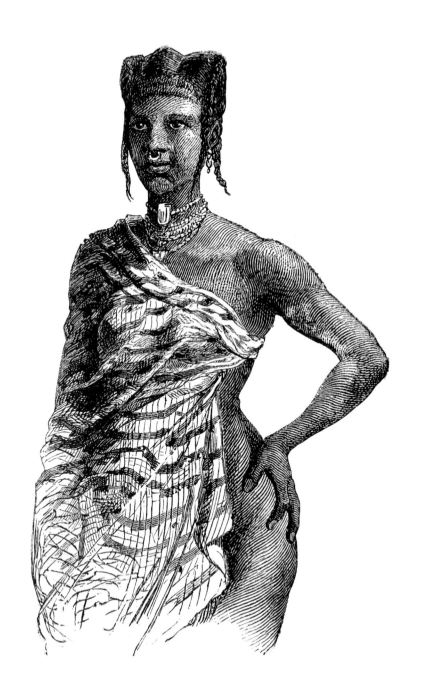

196 Senegal

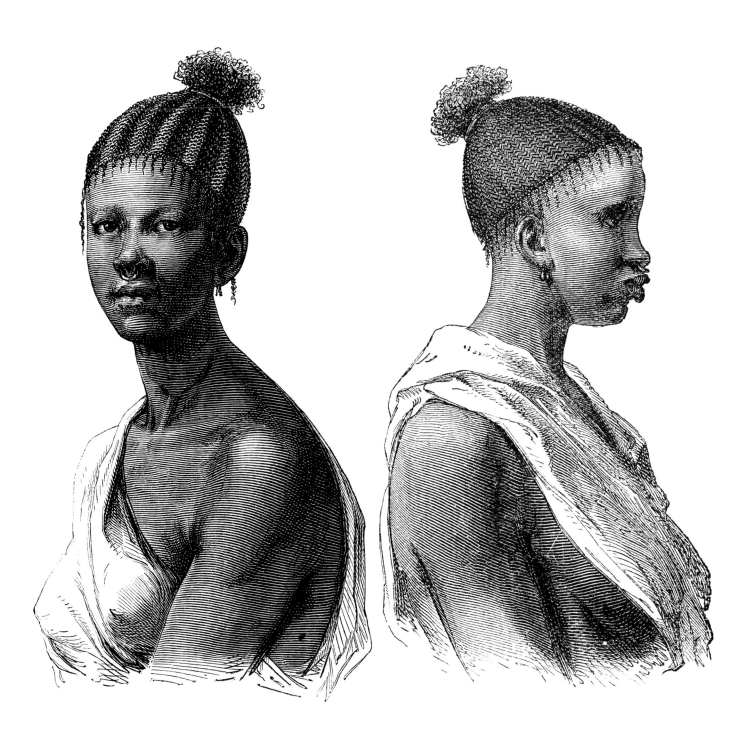

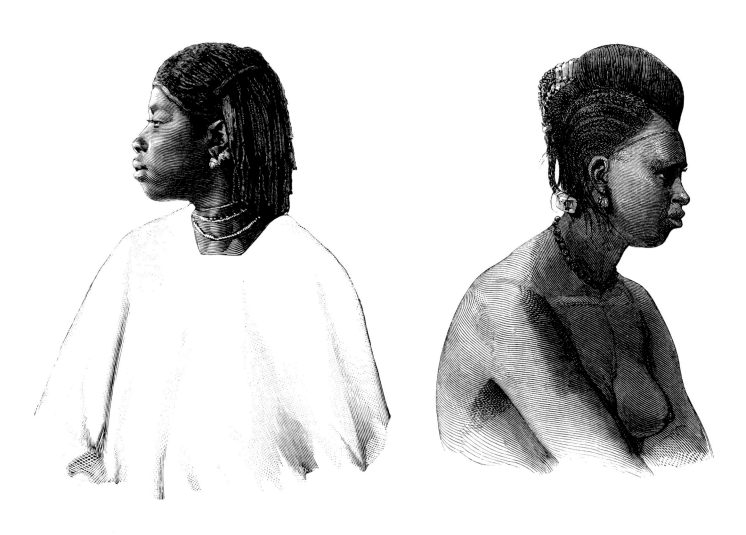

198   Senegal

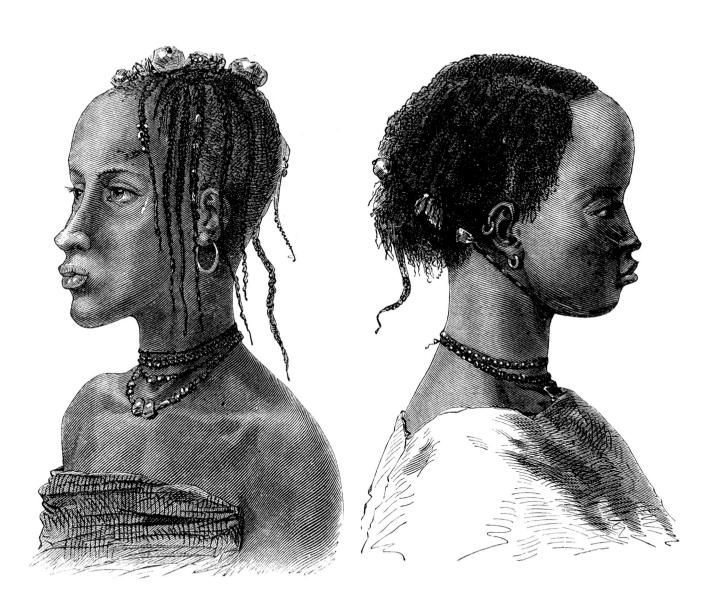

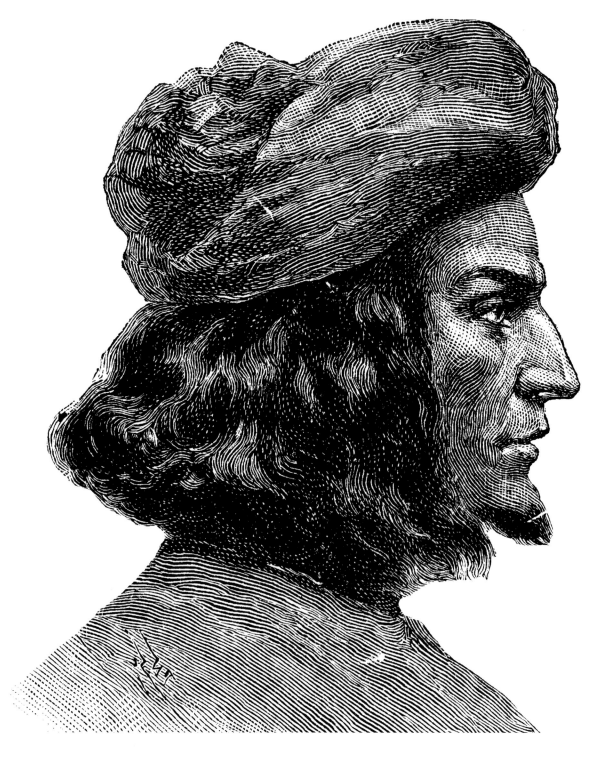

202   Yemen

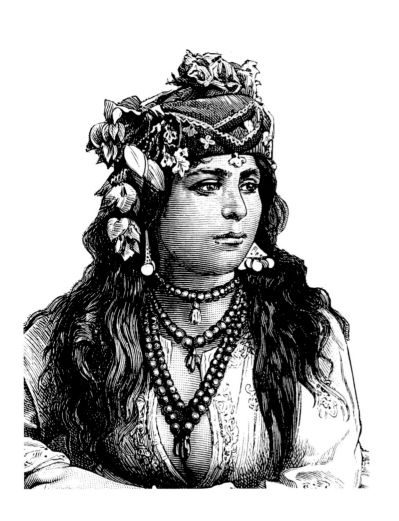
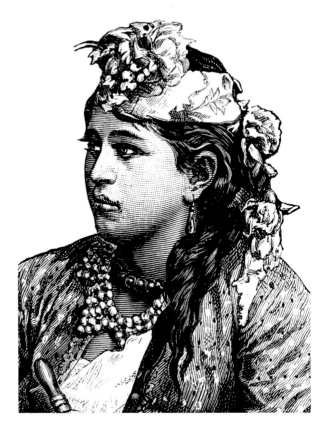

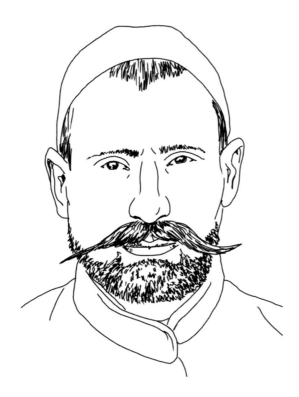

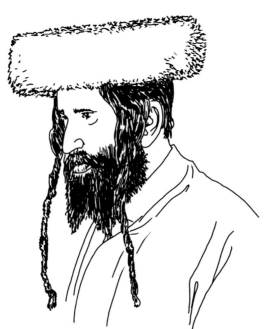

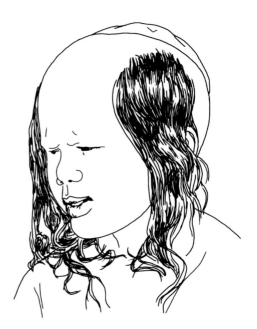

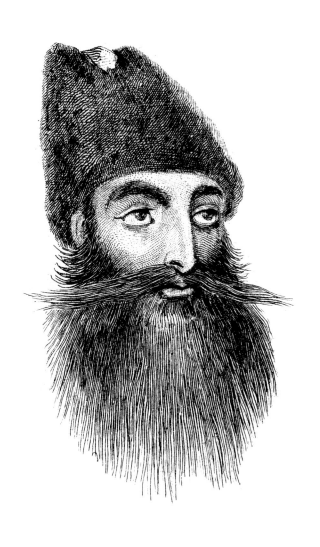

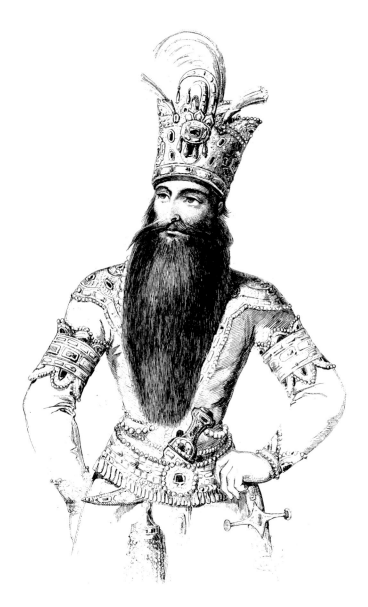

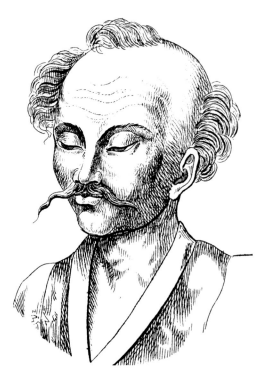

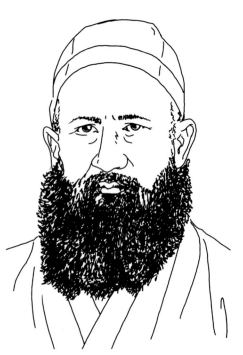

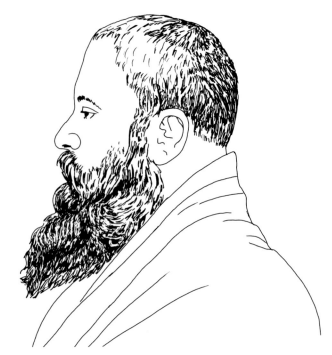

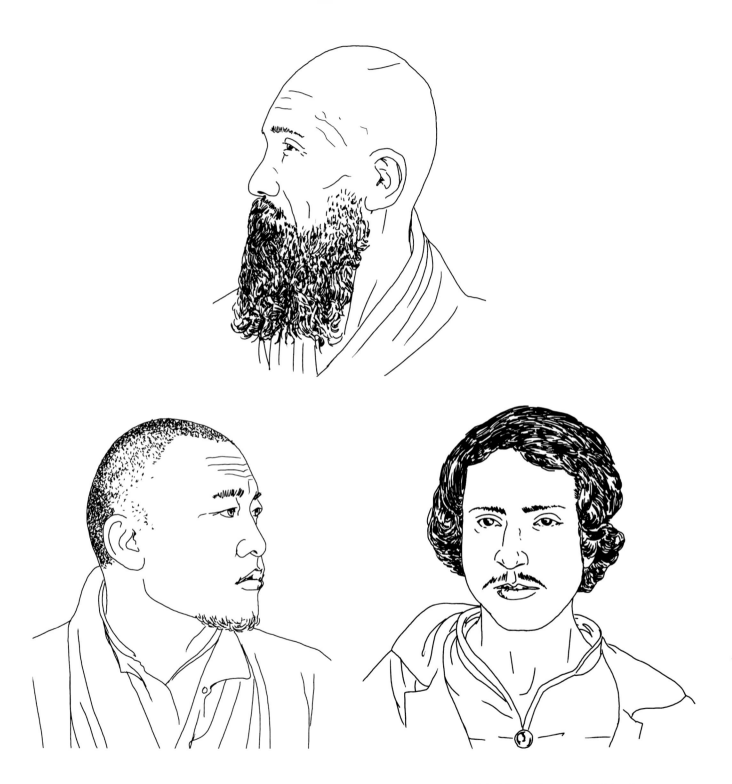

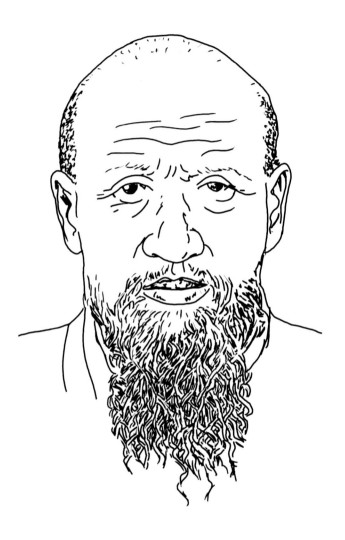

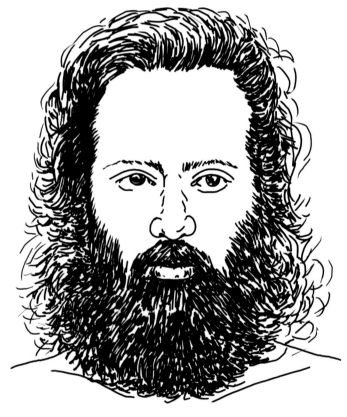

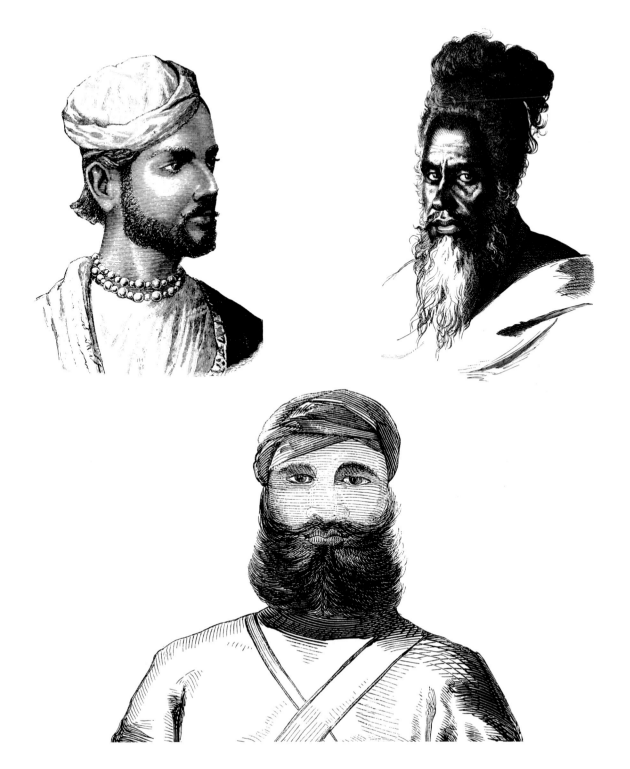

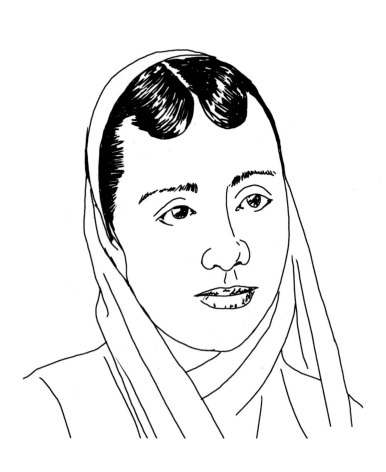
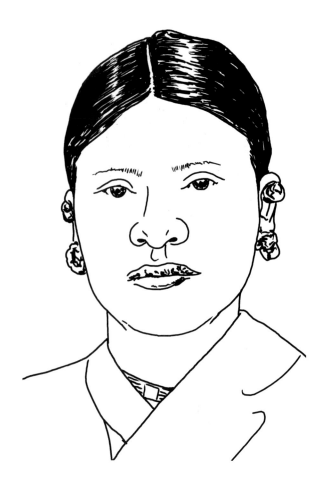

210   Parsi/Hindu, India

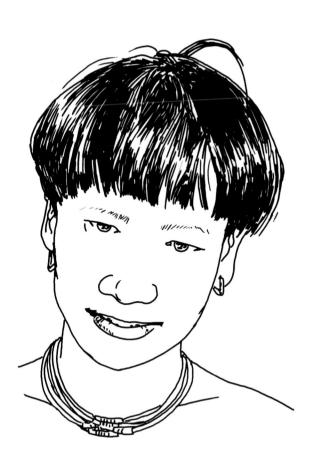
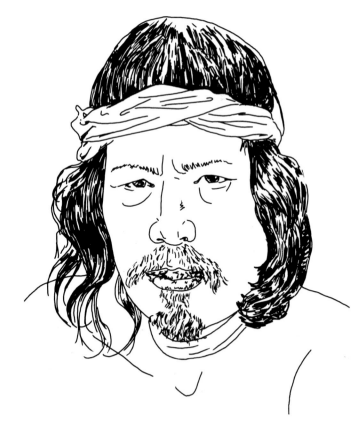

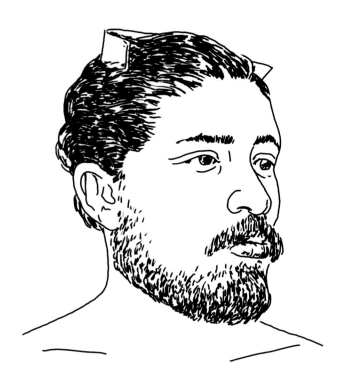

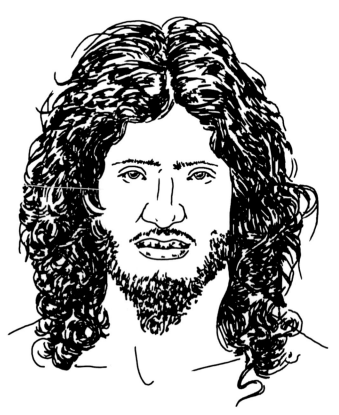

212   Sri Lanka

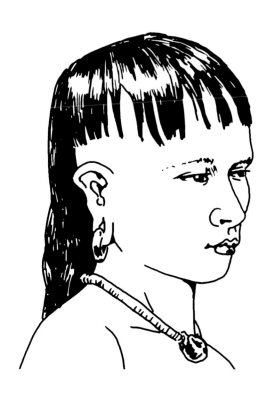

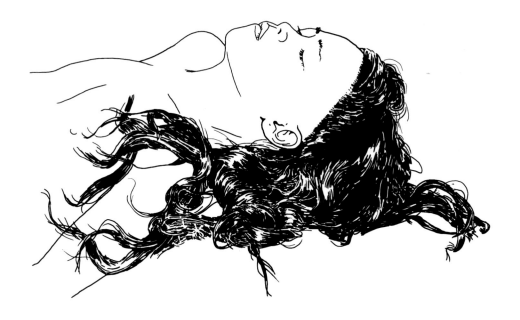

Borneo, Malaysia   213

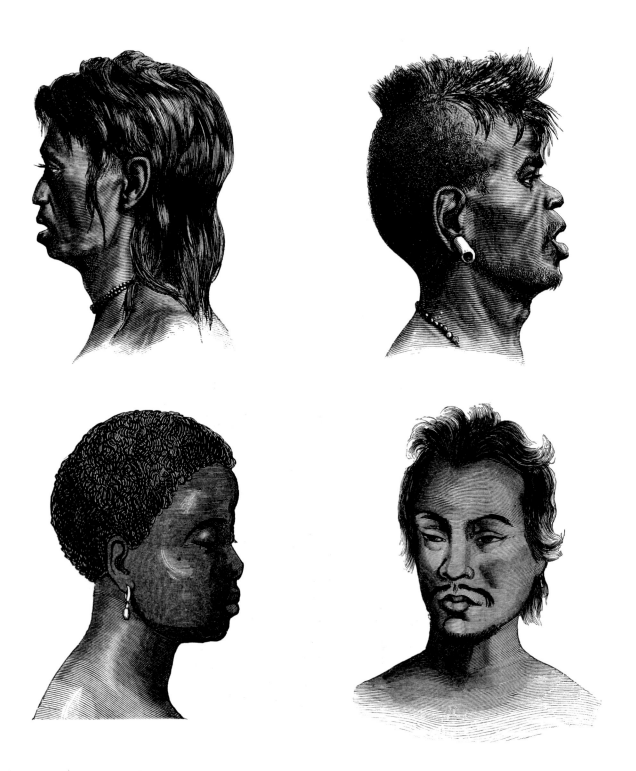

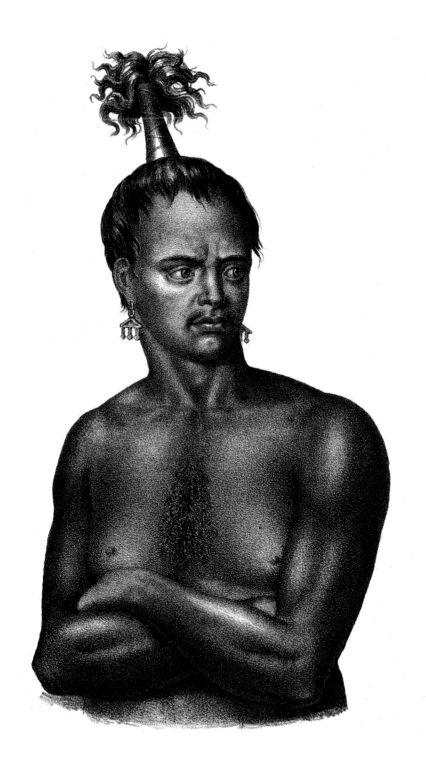

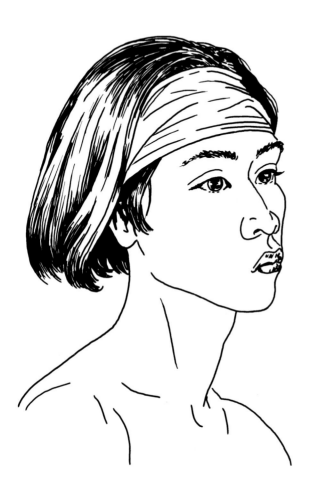
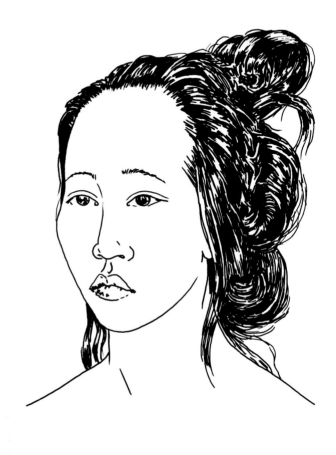

216   Bali, Indonesia

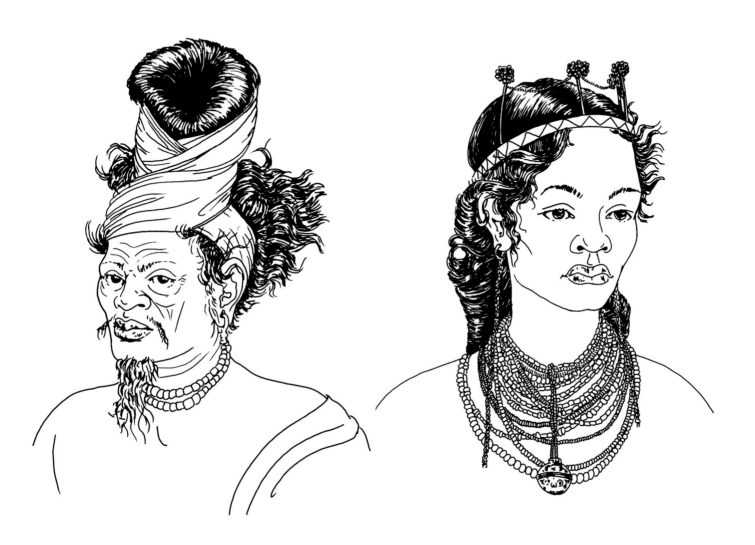

Ceram, Indonesia 217

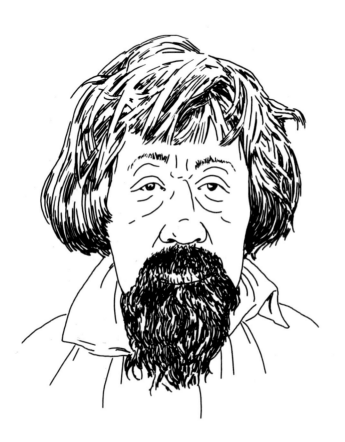

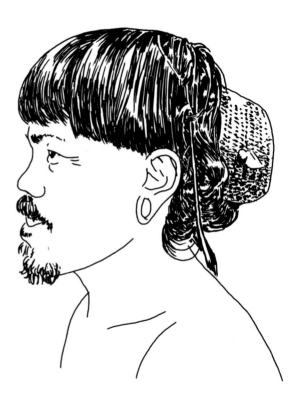

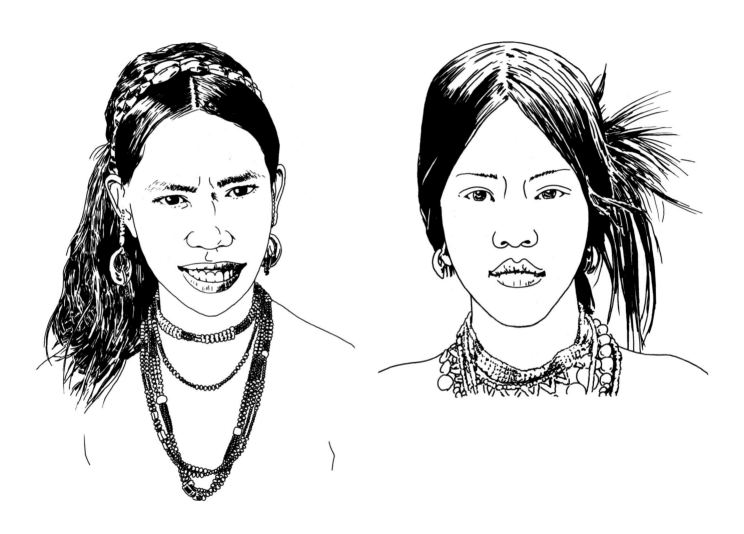

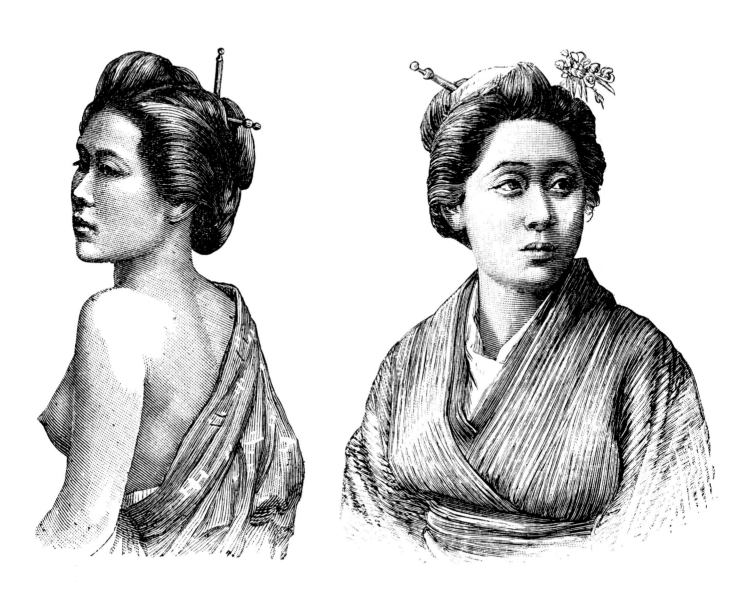

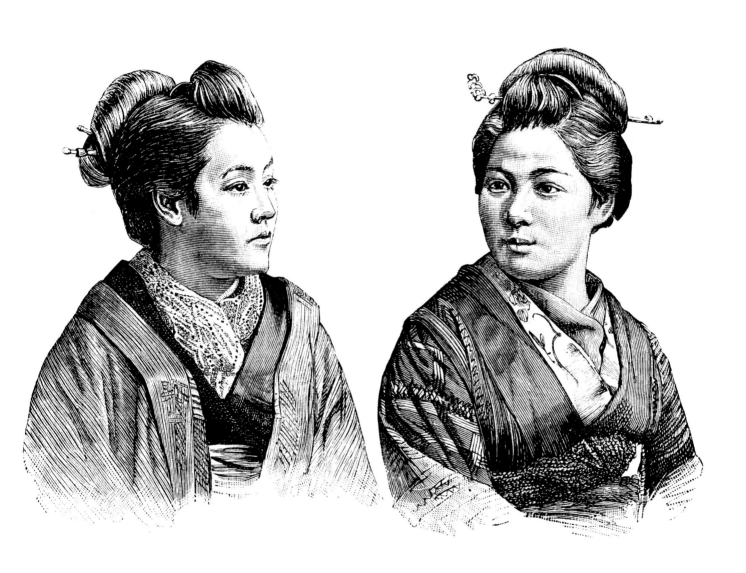

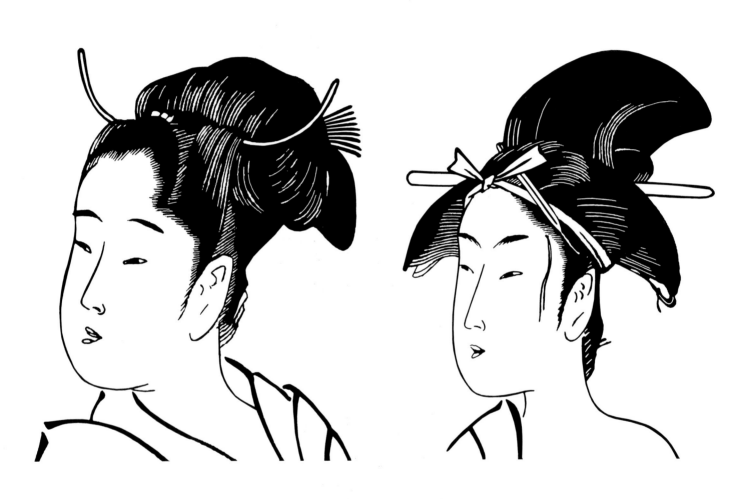

222   Japan

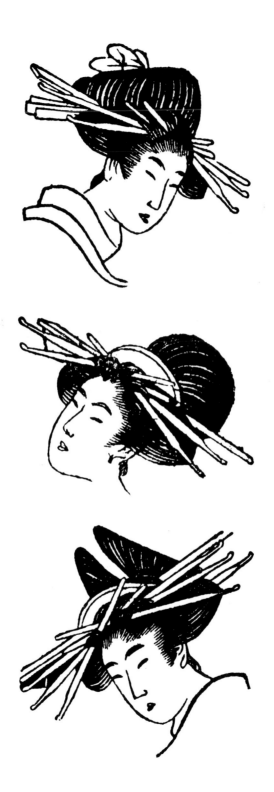

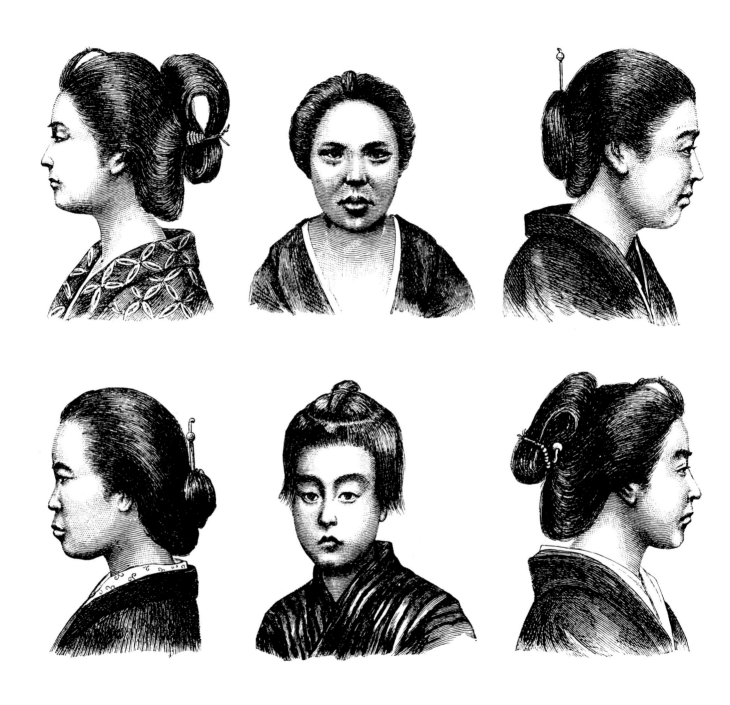

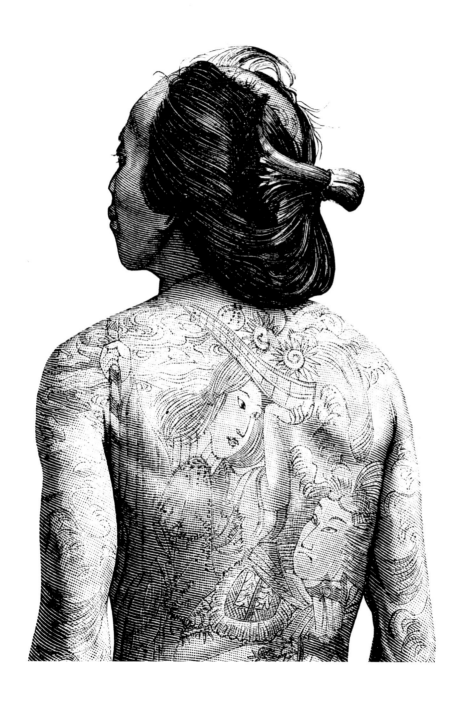

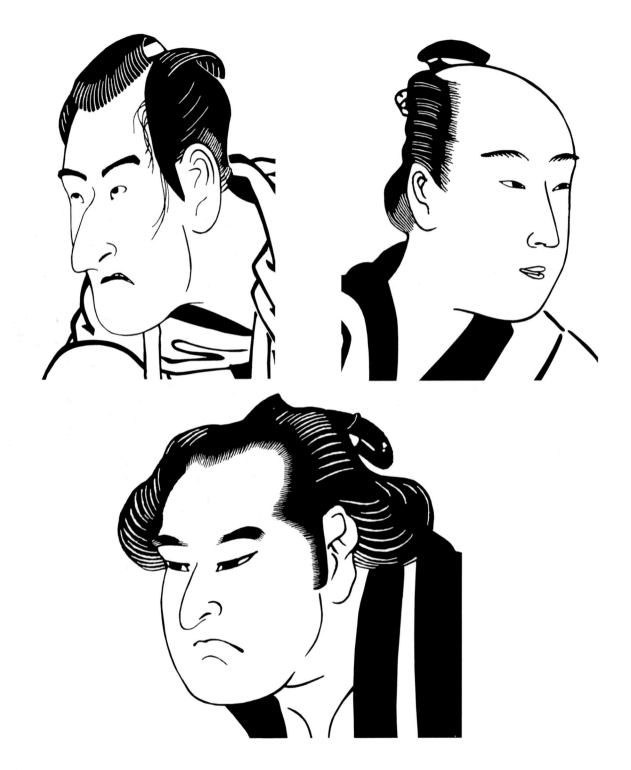

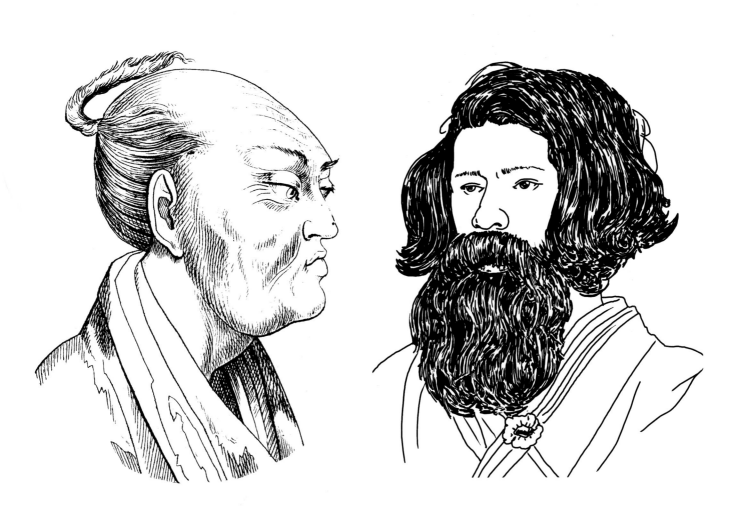

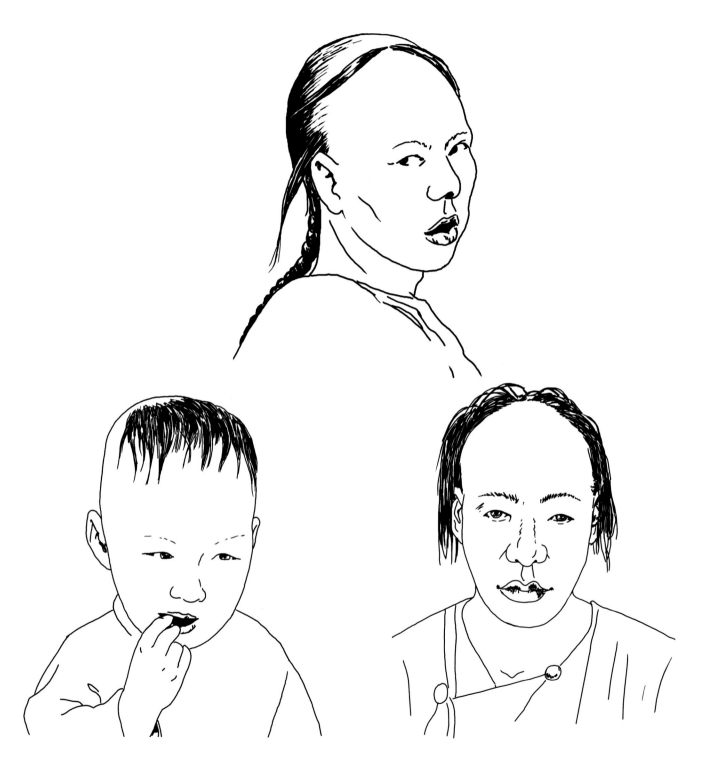

228   China

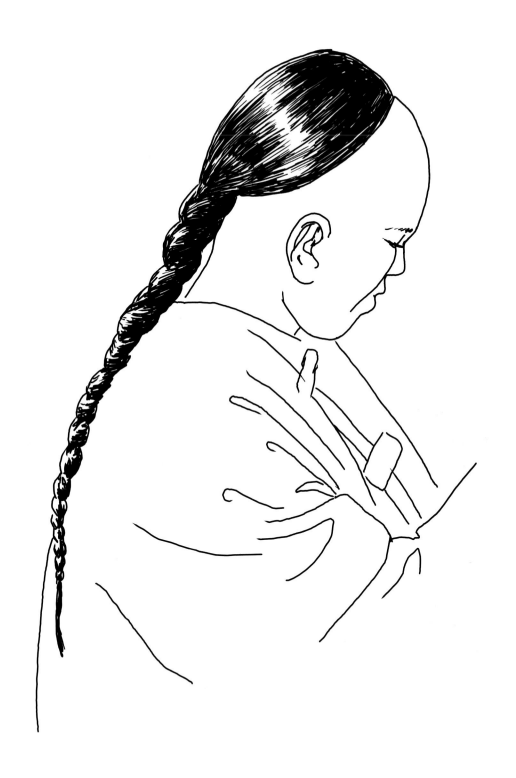

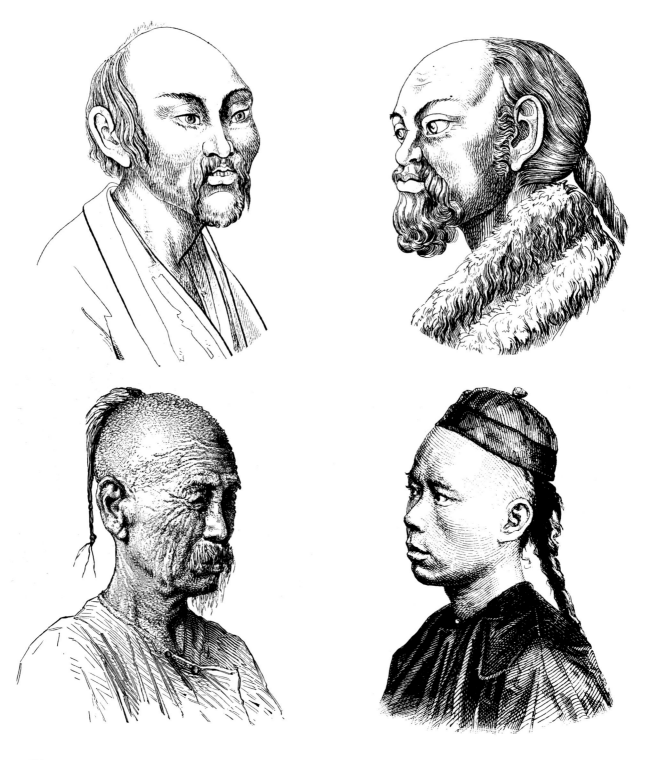

230   China

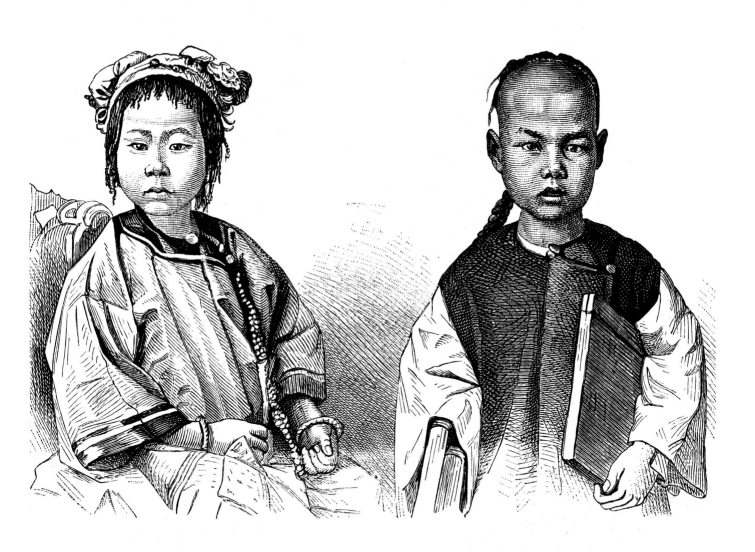

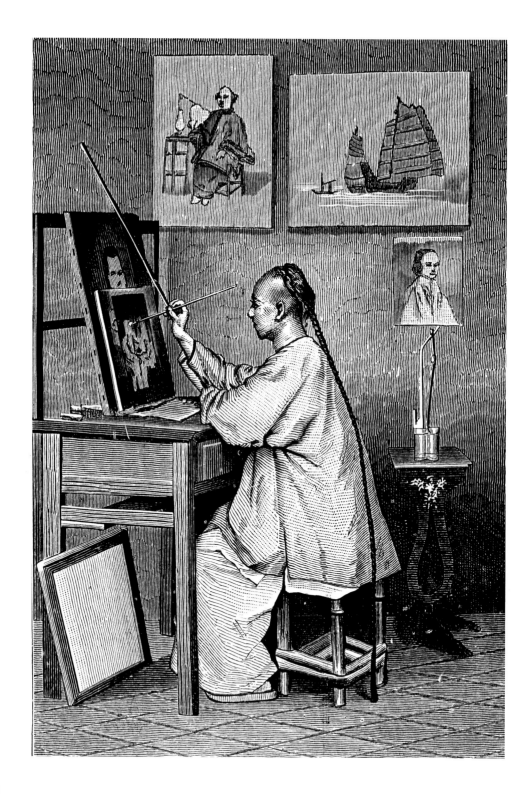

232   China

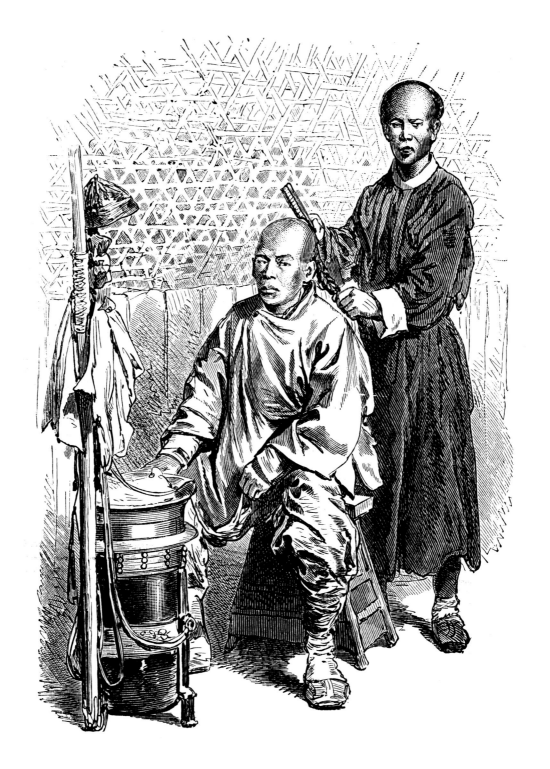

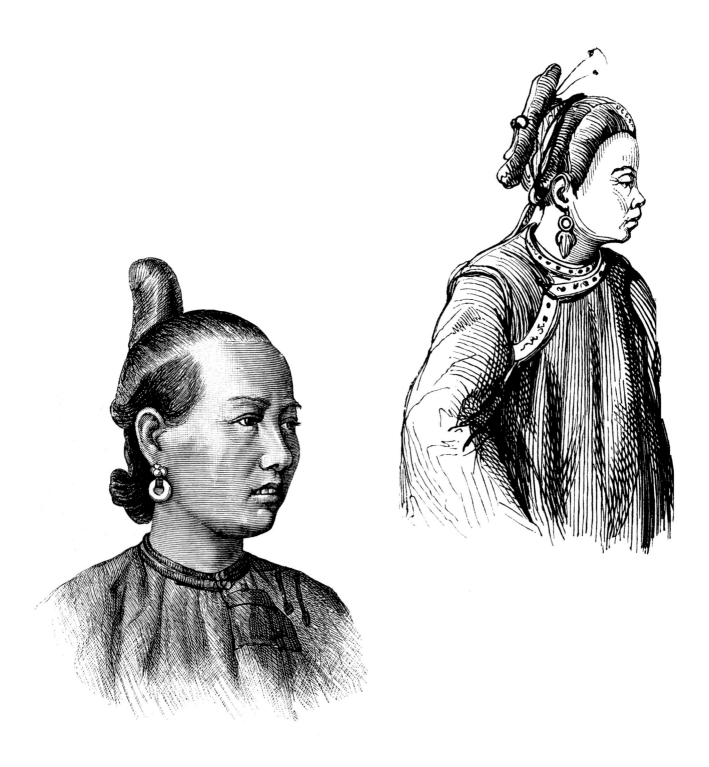

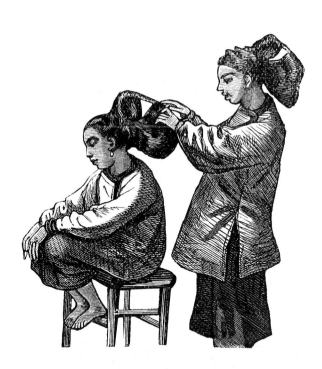

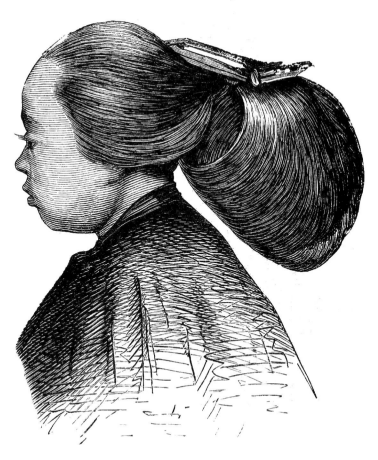

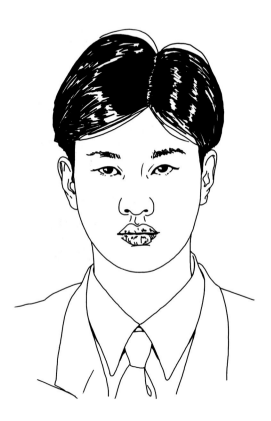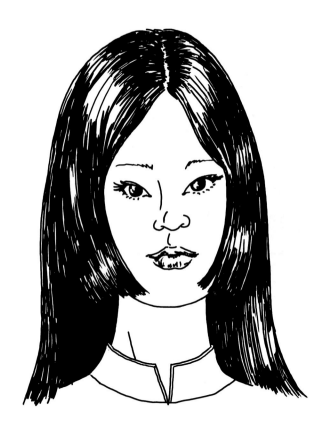

236   Chinese, 1970s

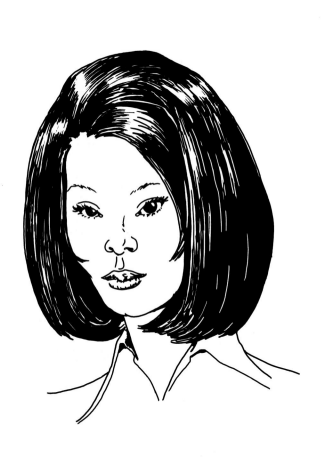

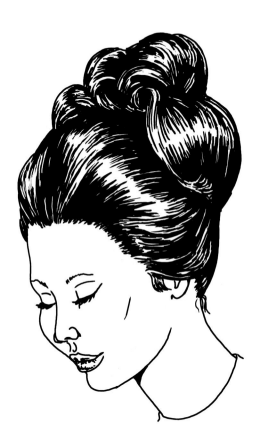

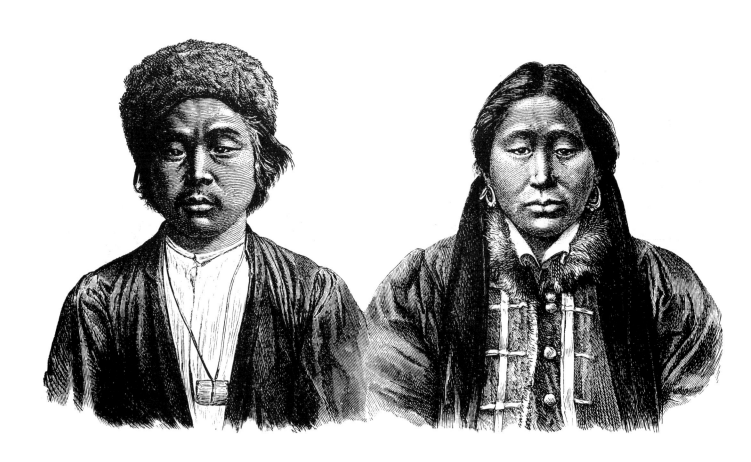

238   Kalmukya

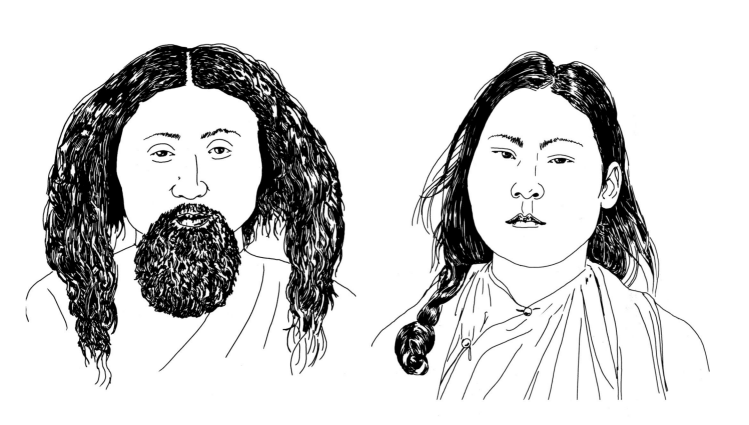

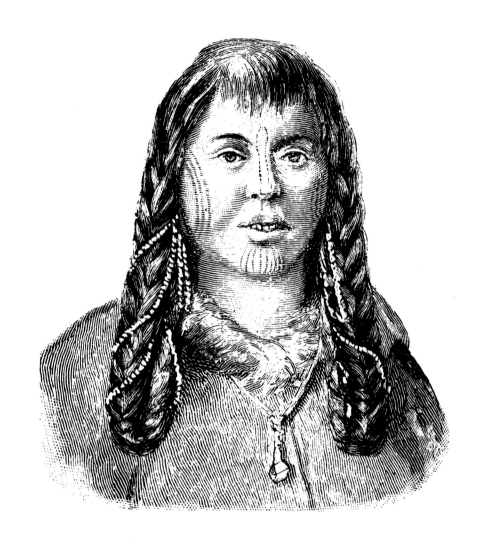

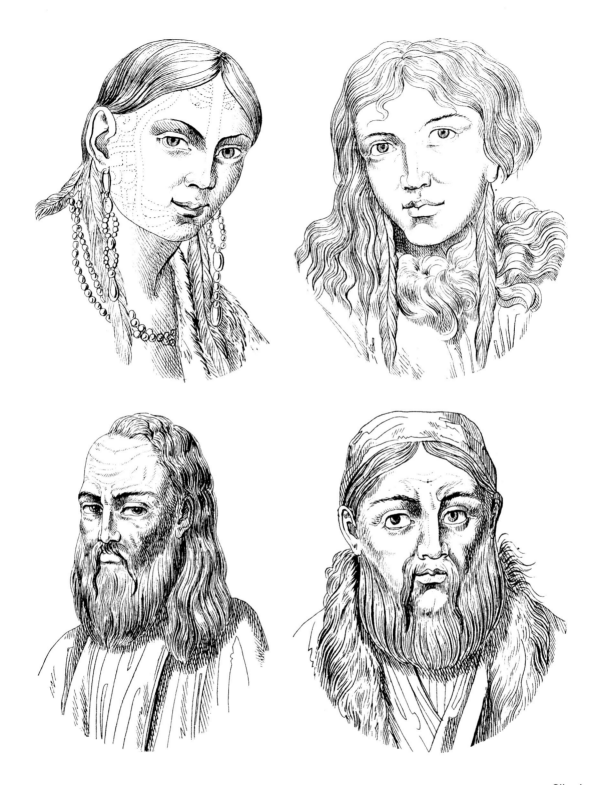

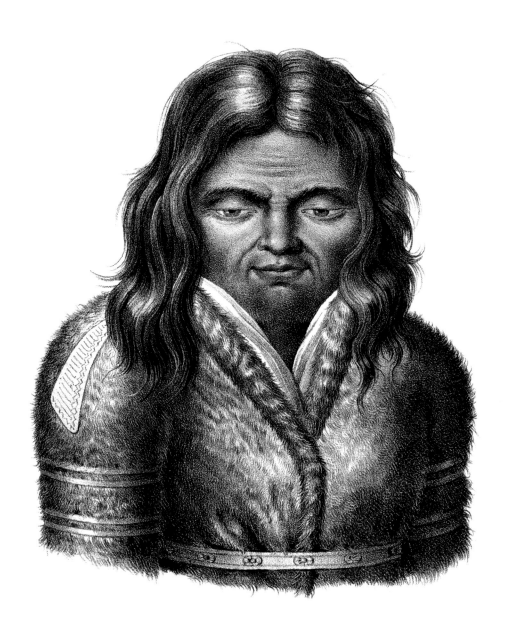

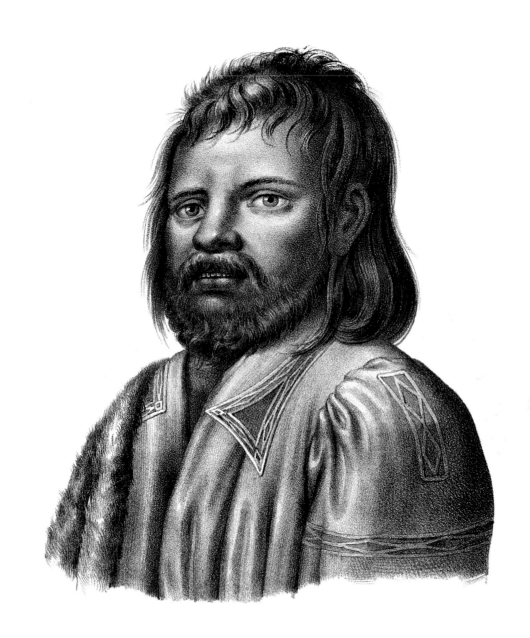

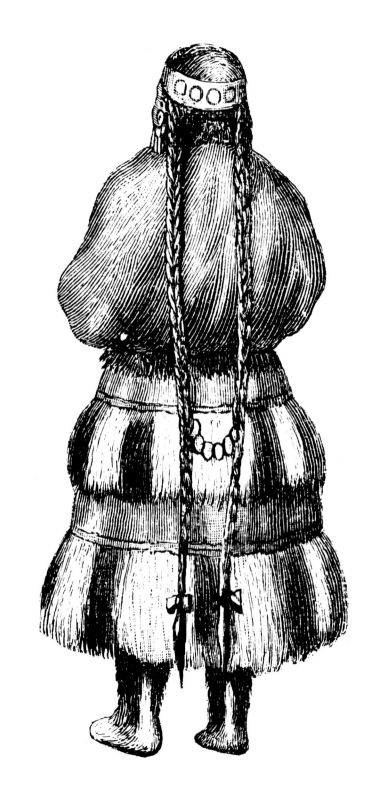

244   Siberia

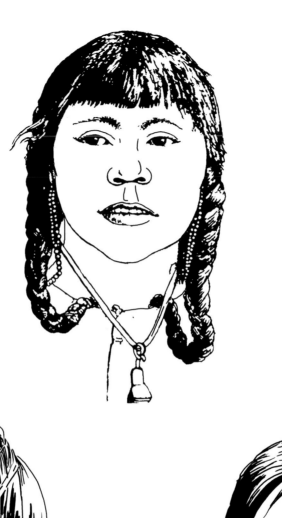
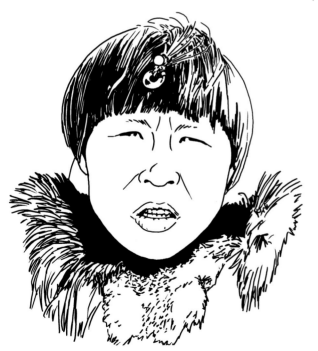
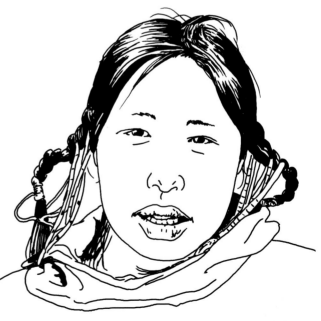

Chuckchee, Siberia 245

AMERICA

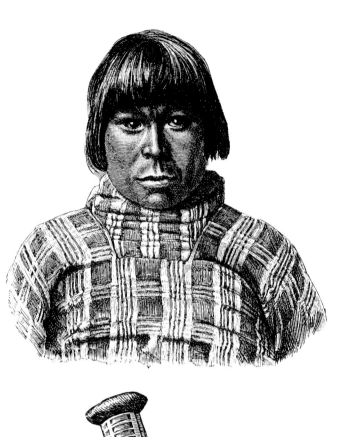

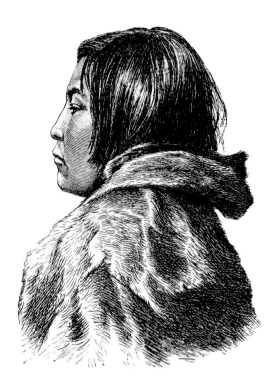

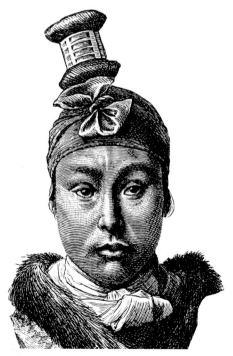

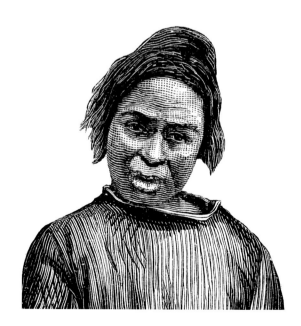

248   Inuit, Canada

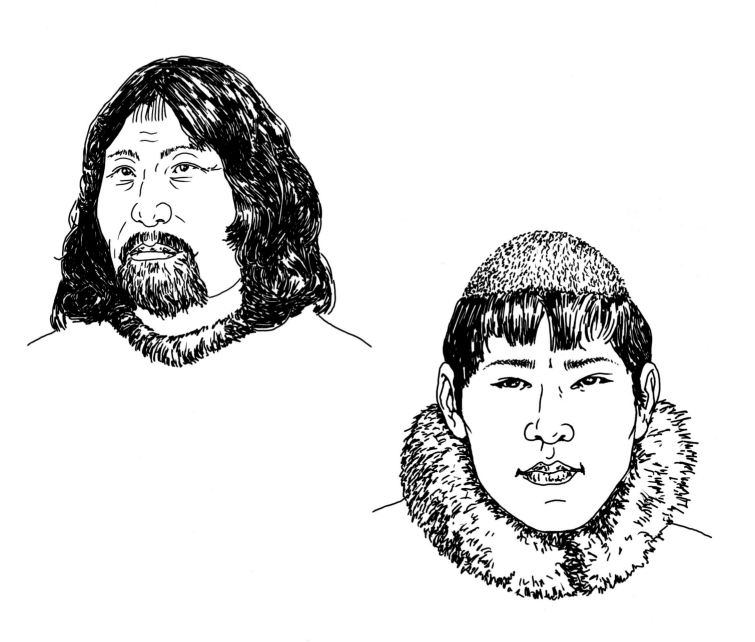

Inuit, Canada   249

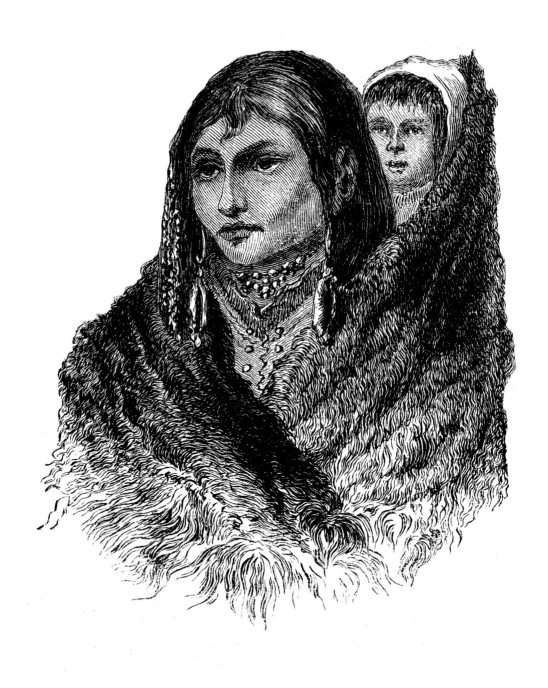

250   Native Americans, USA

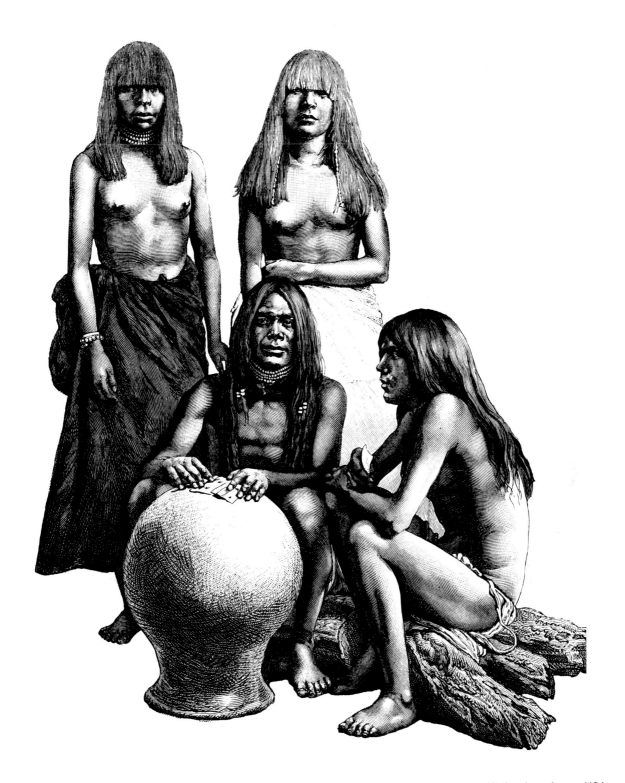

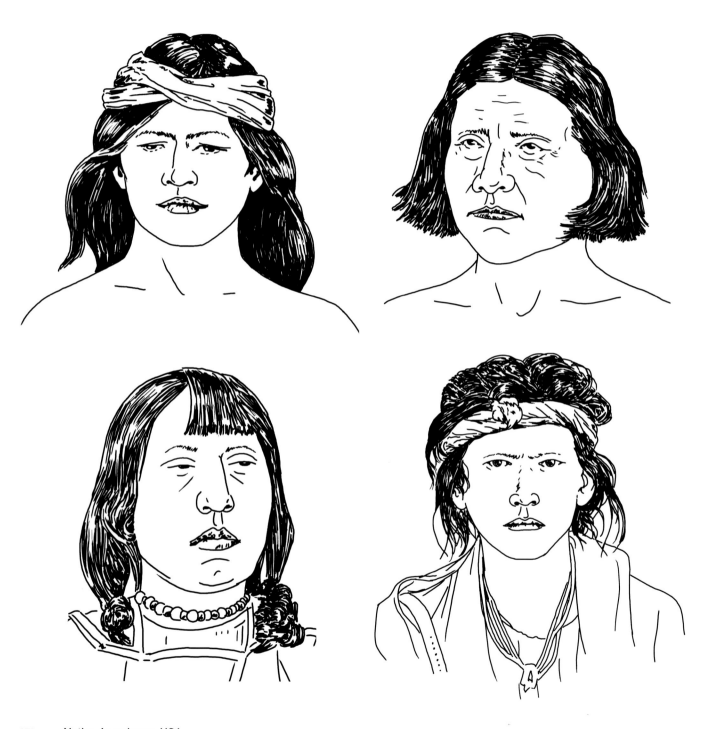

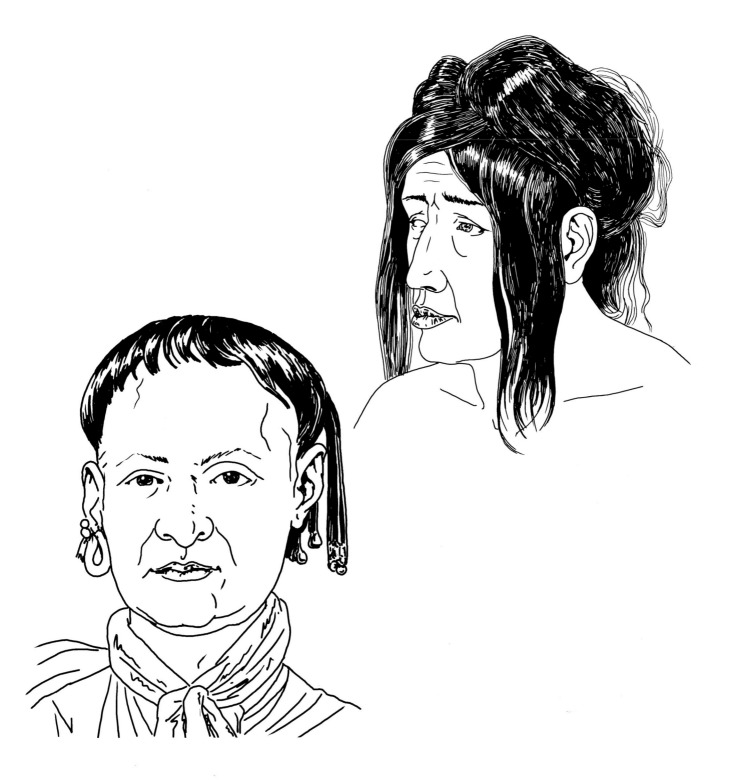

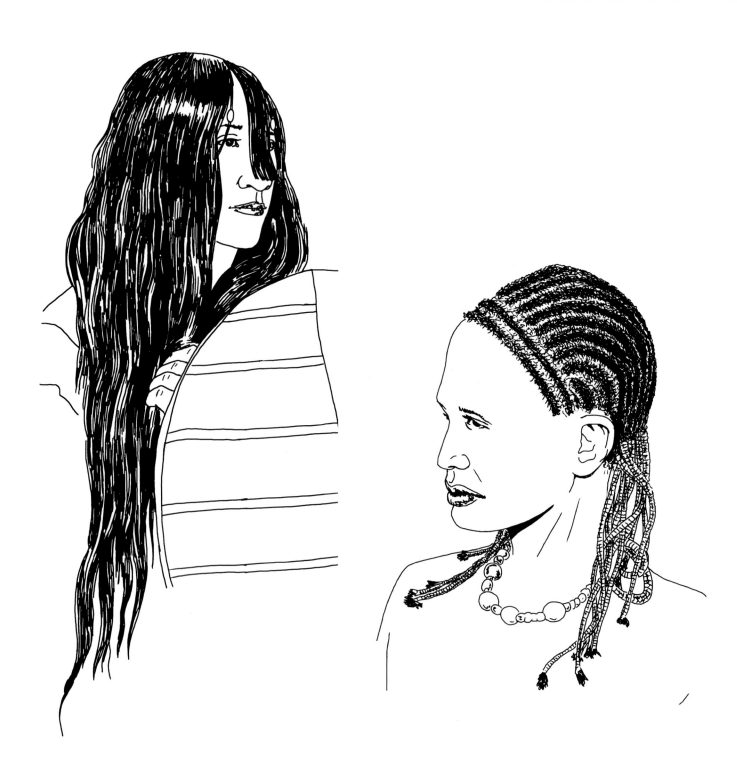

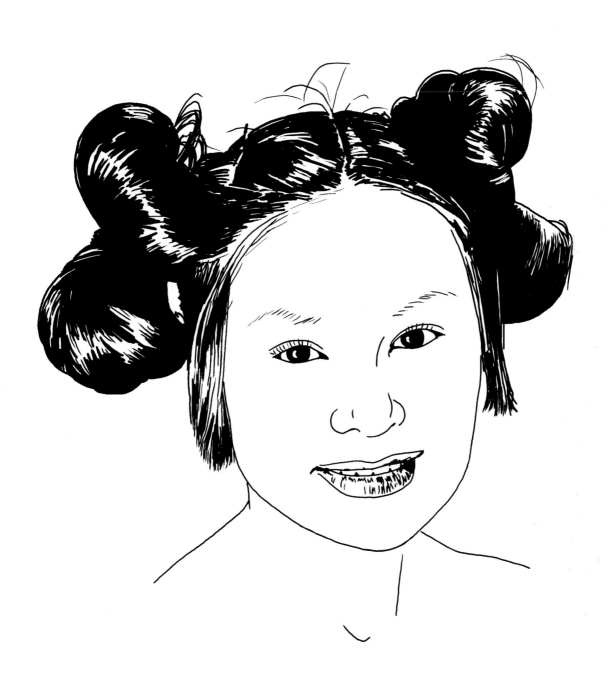

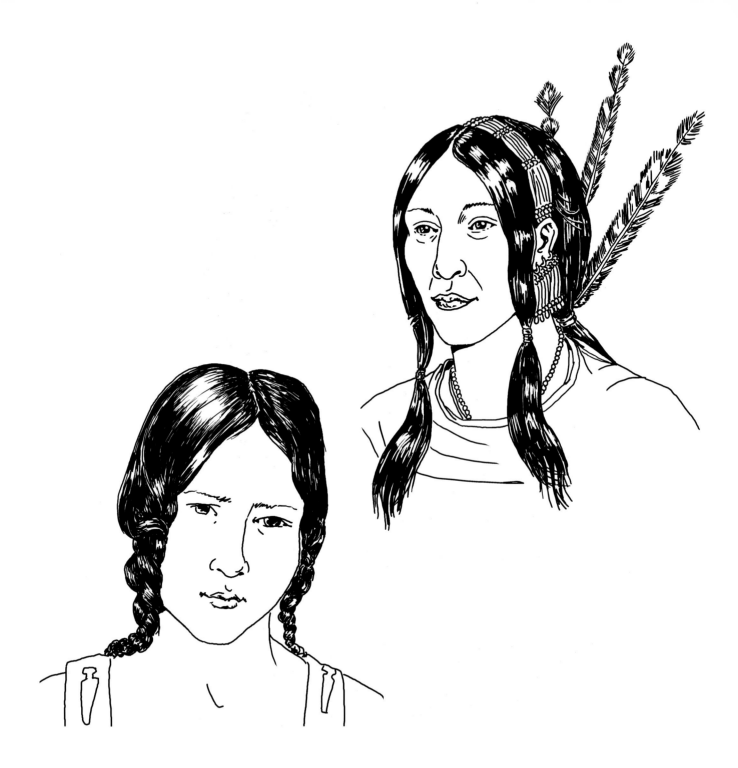

256   Native Americans, USA

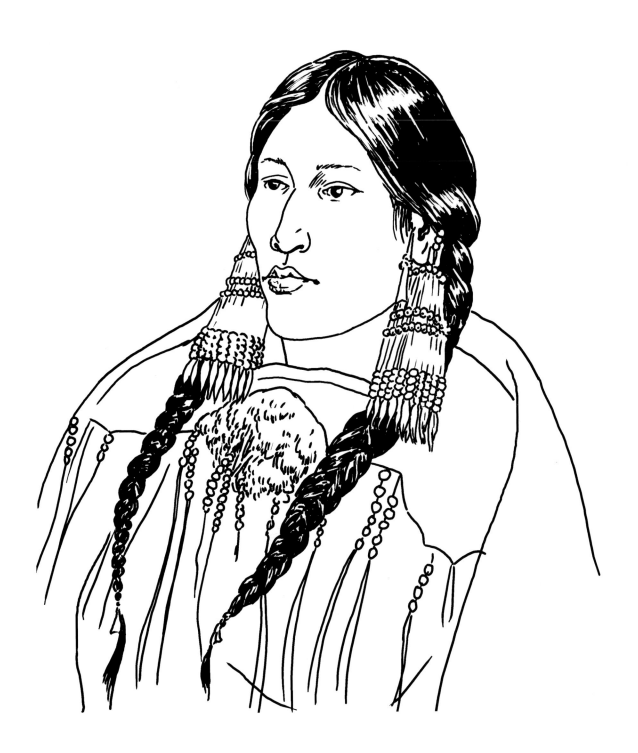

Native Americans, USA   257

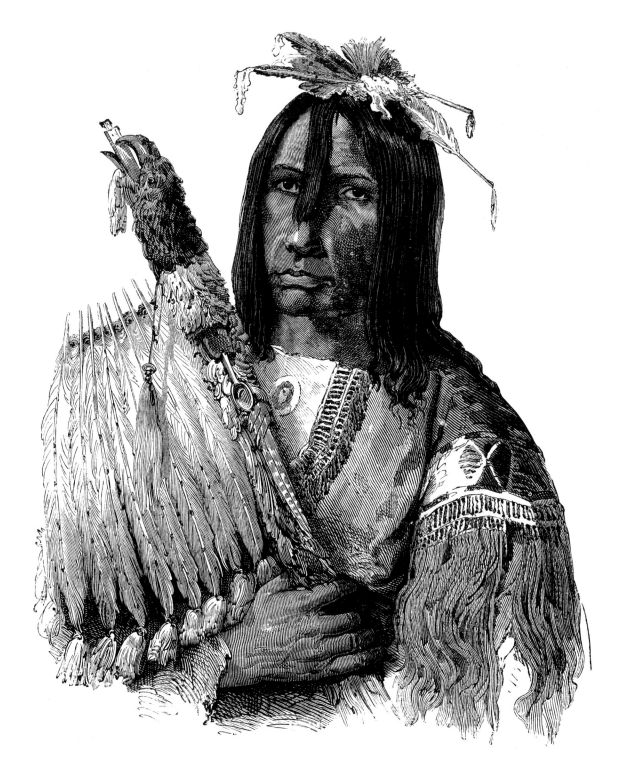

258   Native Americans, USA

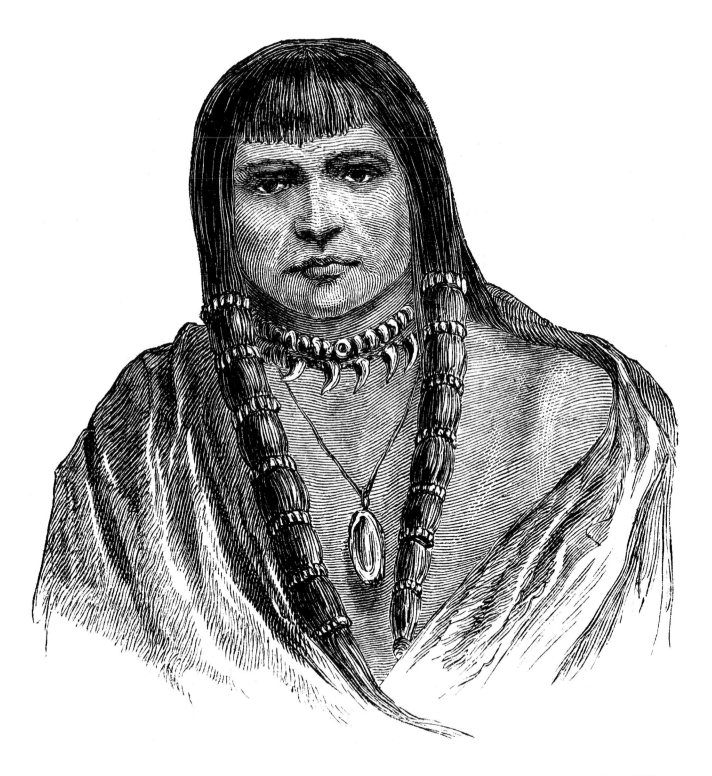

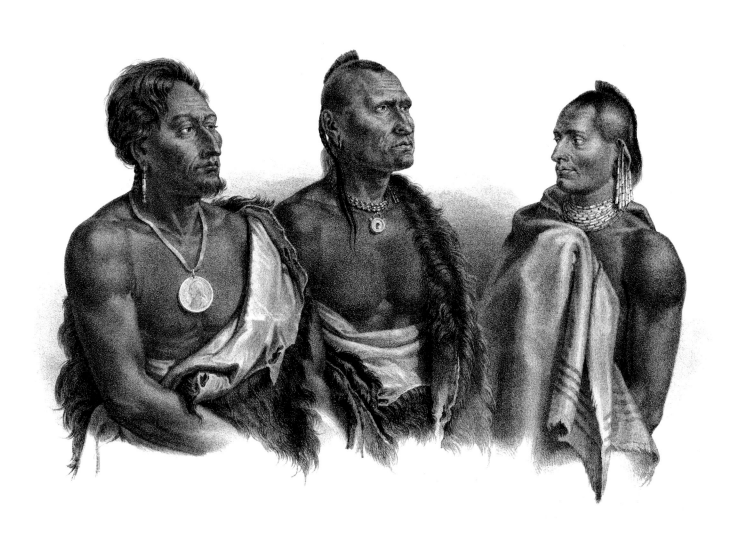

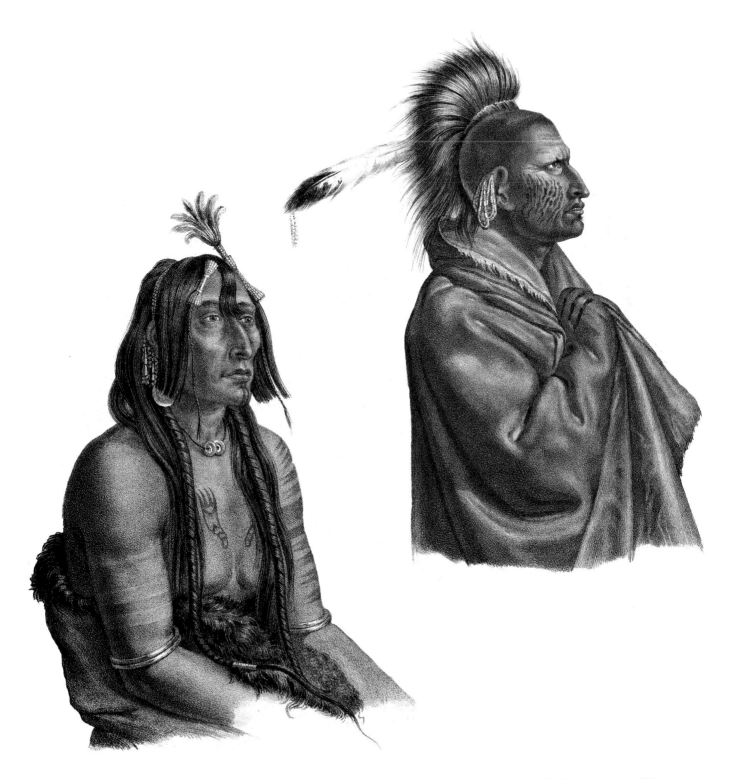

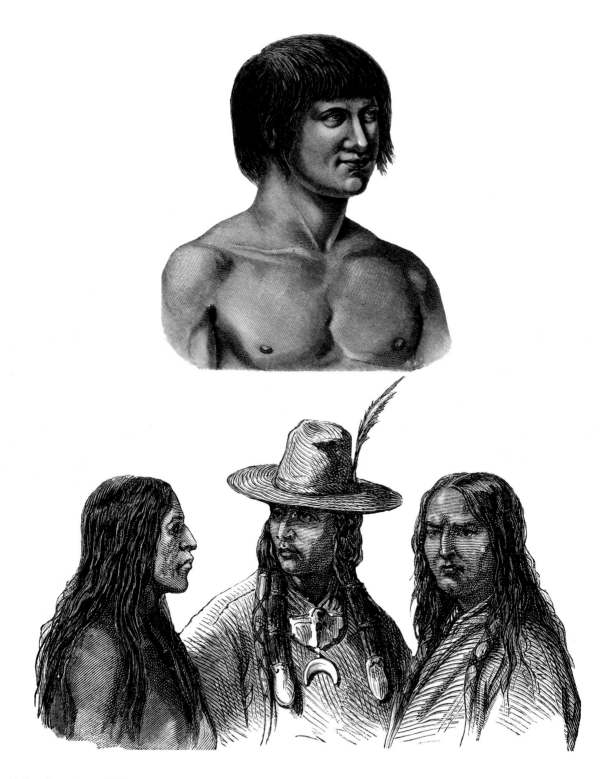

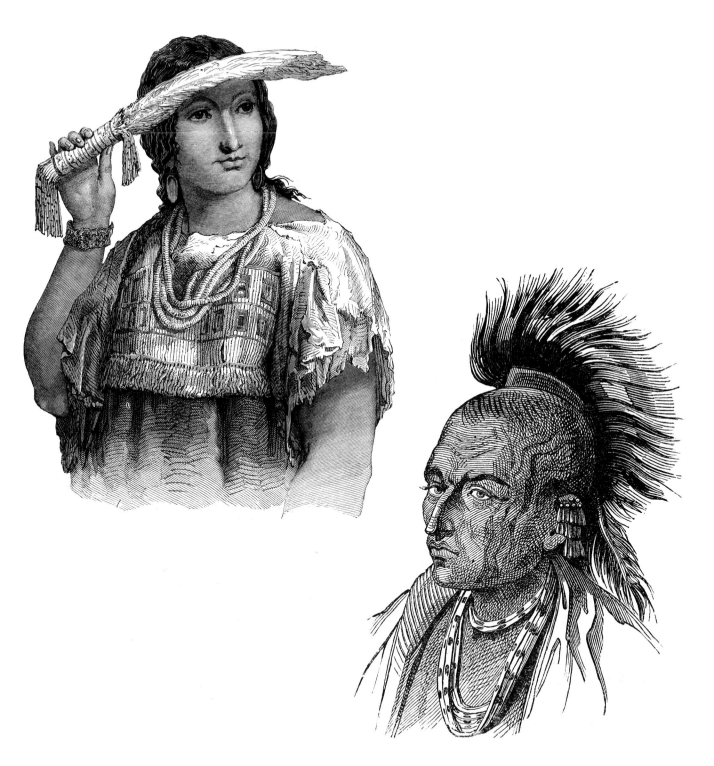

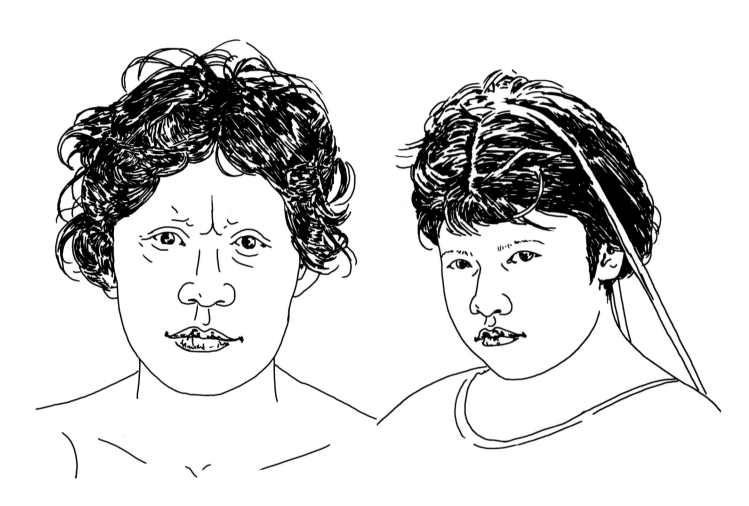

264   Costa Rica

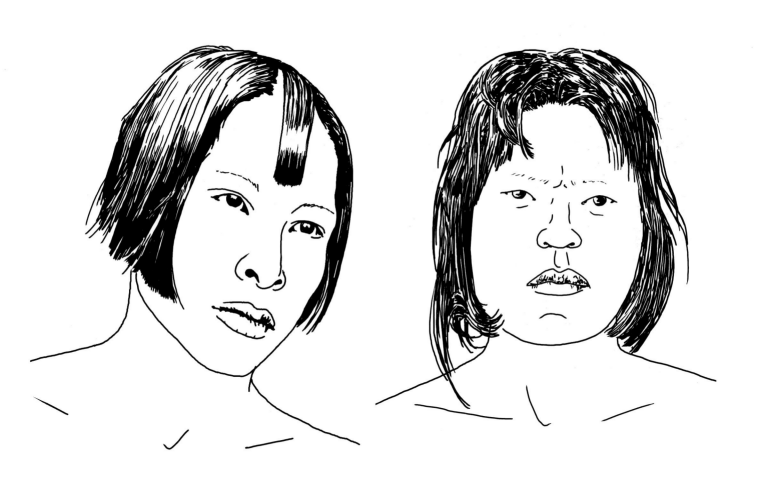

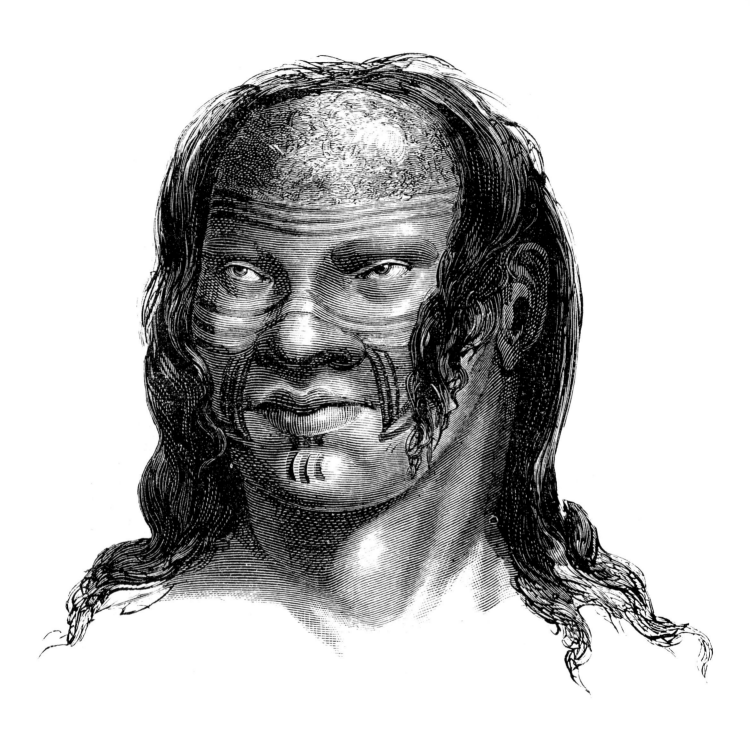

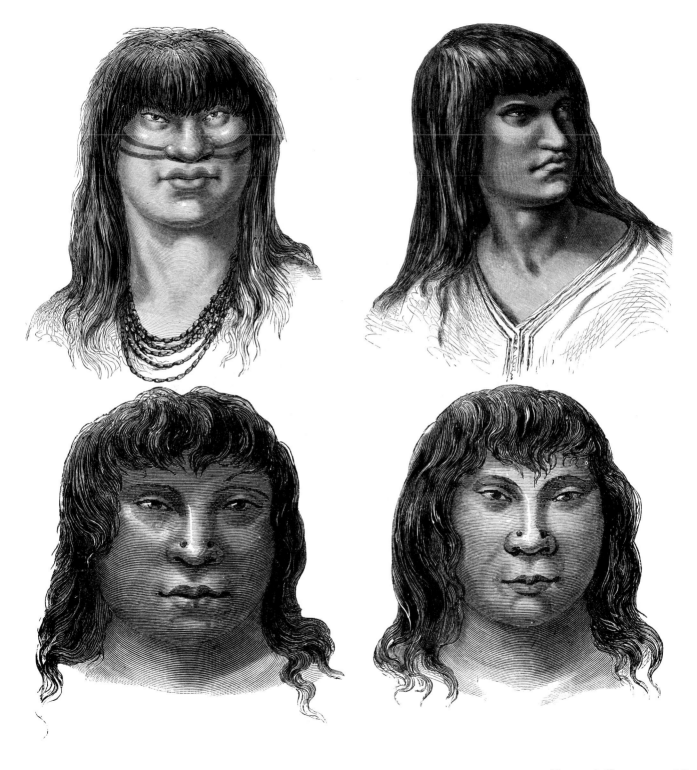

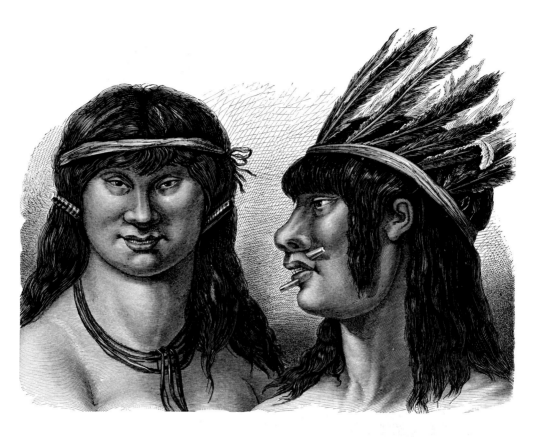

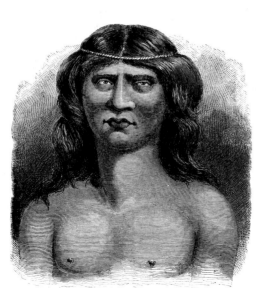

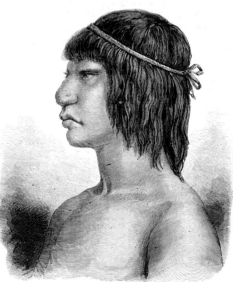

Venezuela/Guyana

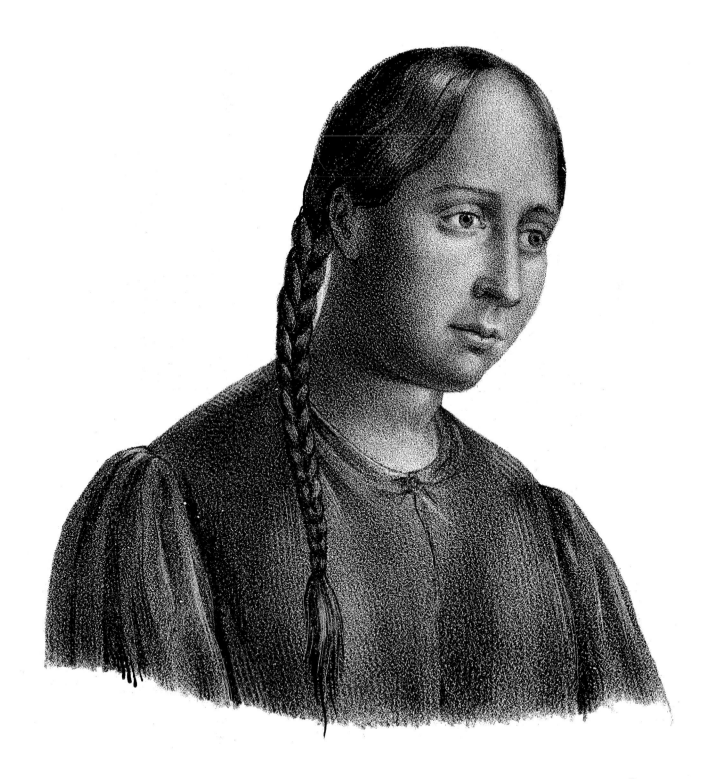

Peru   269

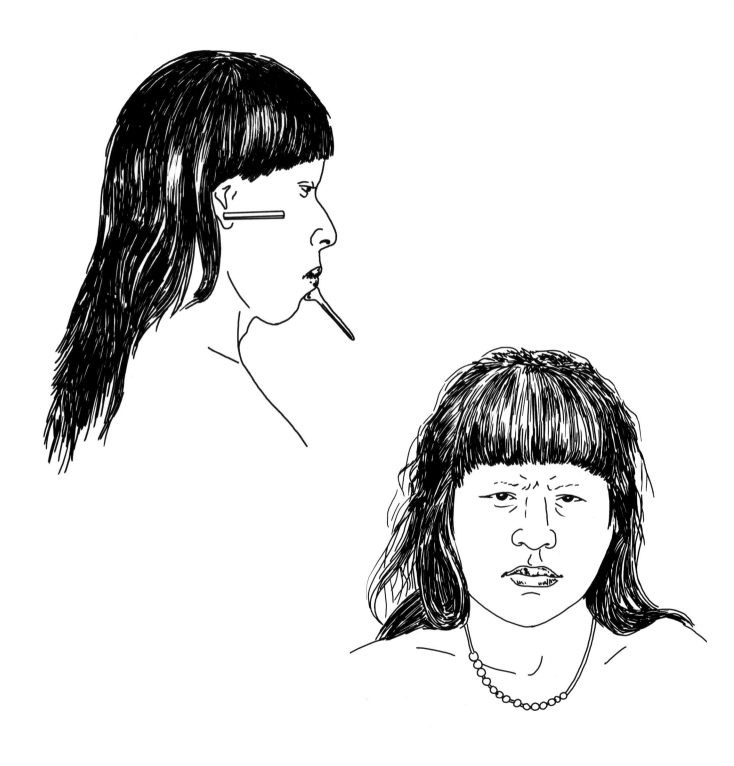

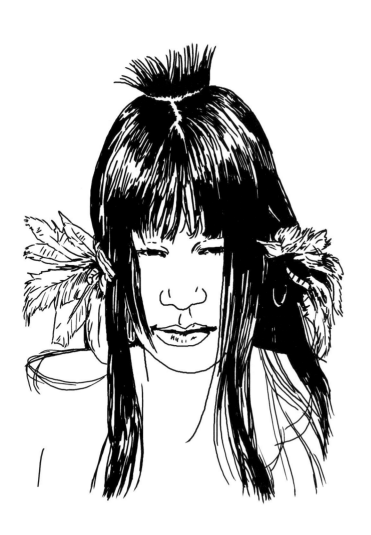
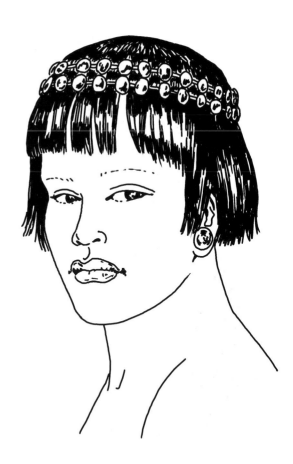

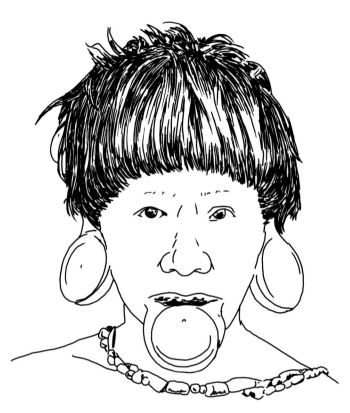

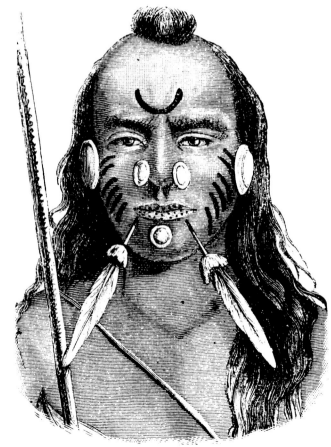

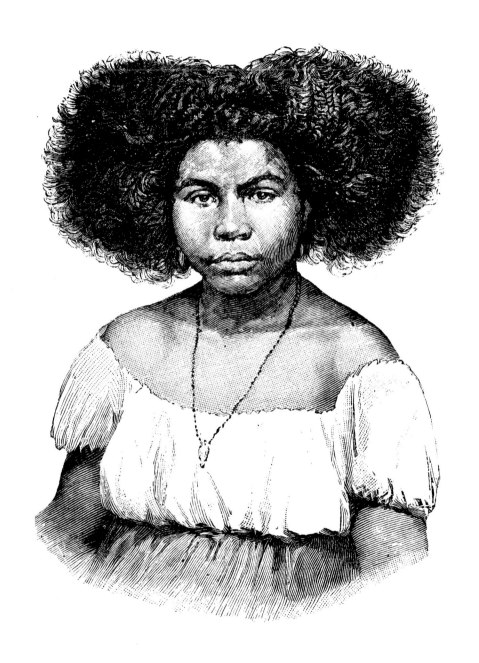

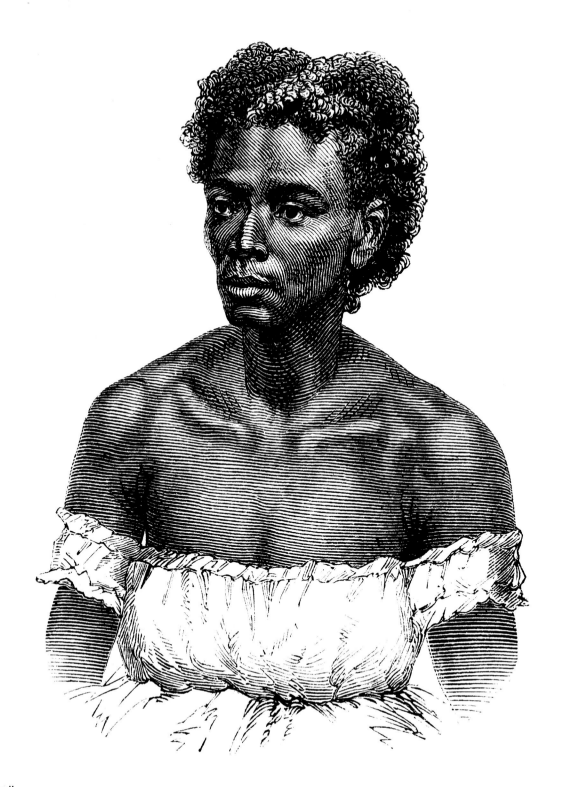

274   Brazil

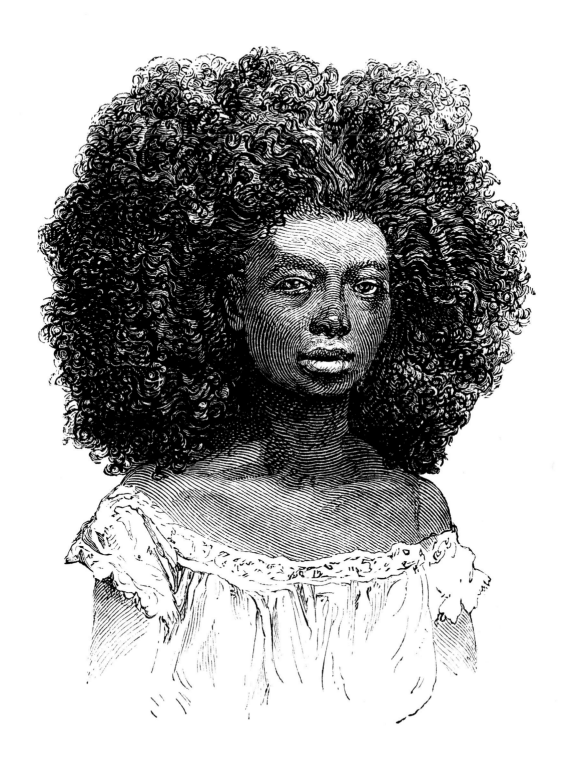

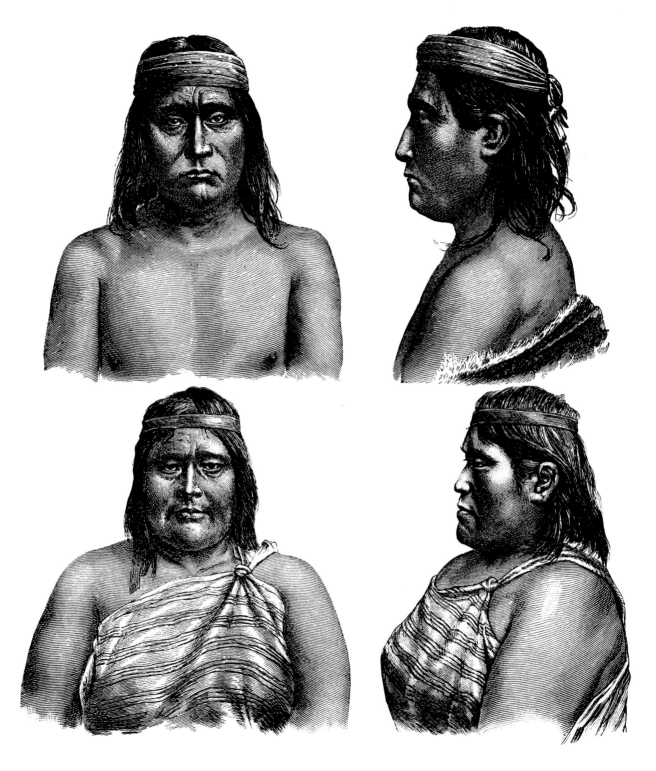

276   Patagonia, Argentina

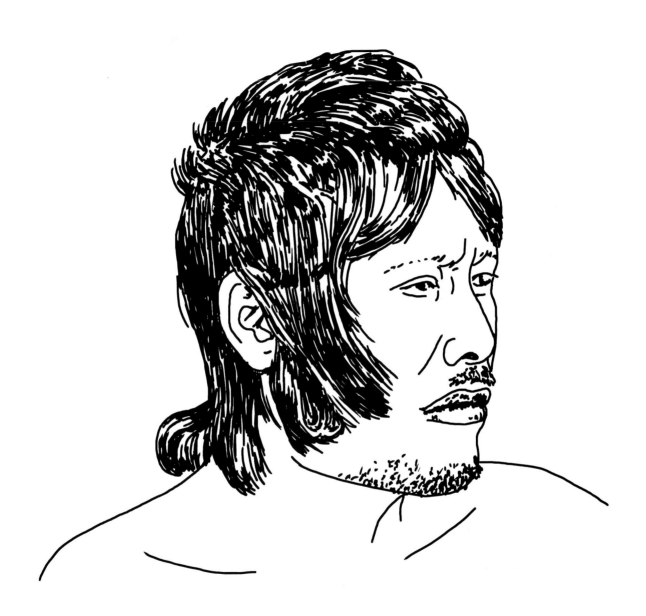

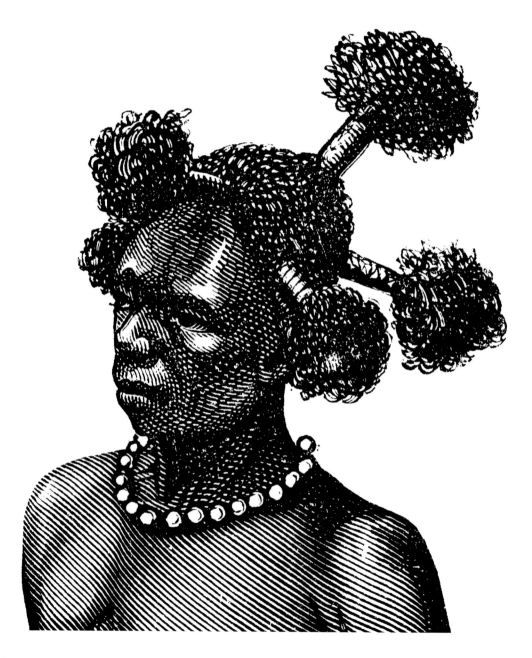

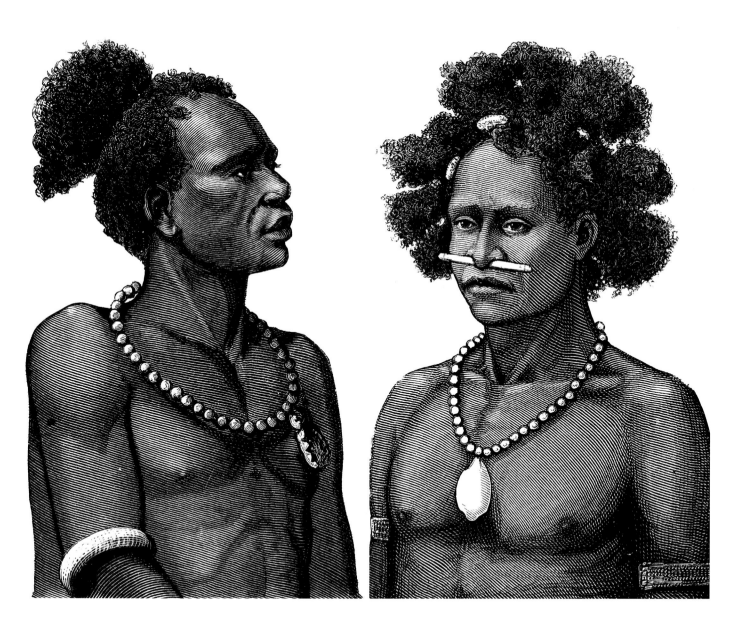

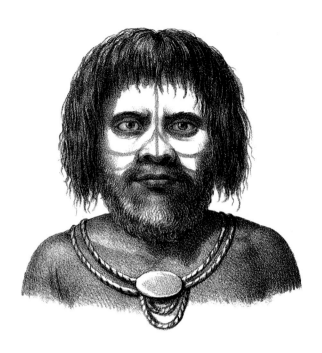

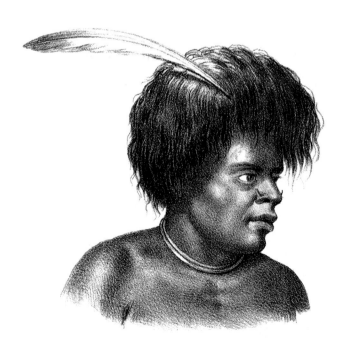

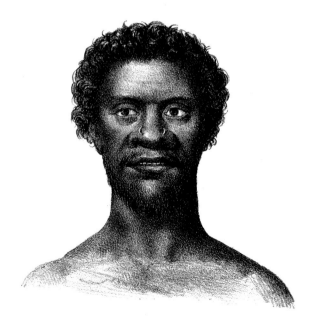

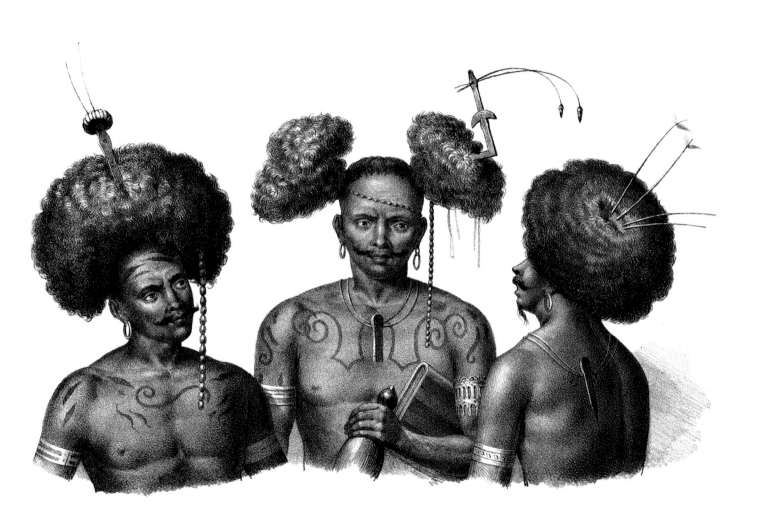

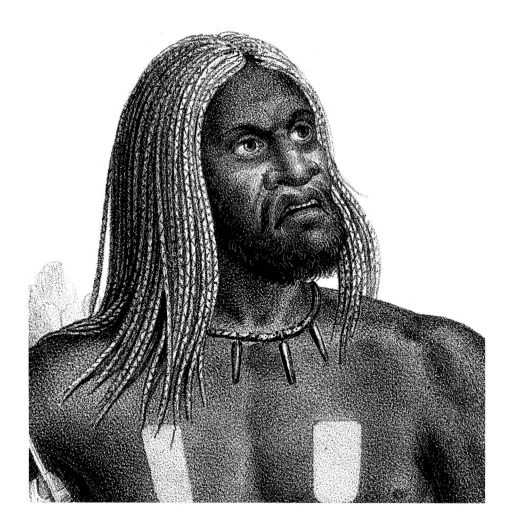

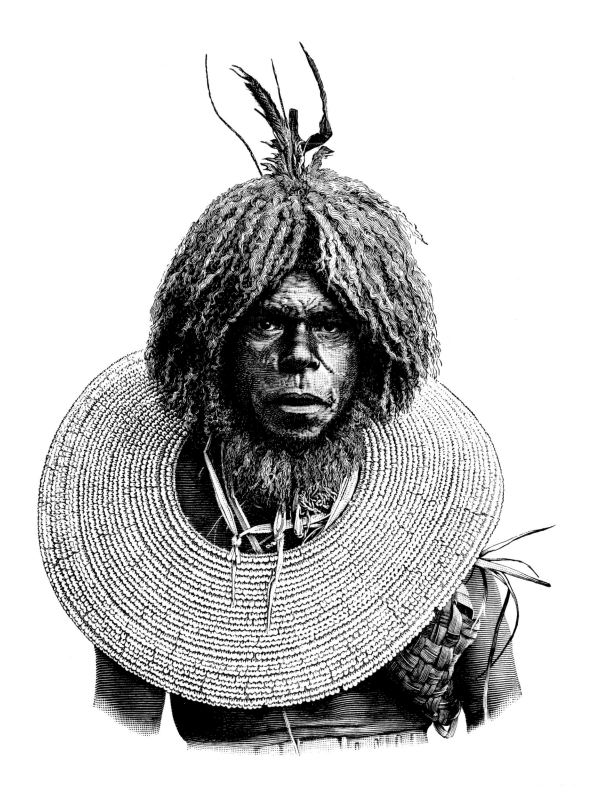

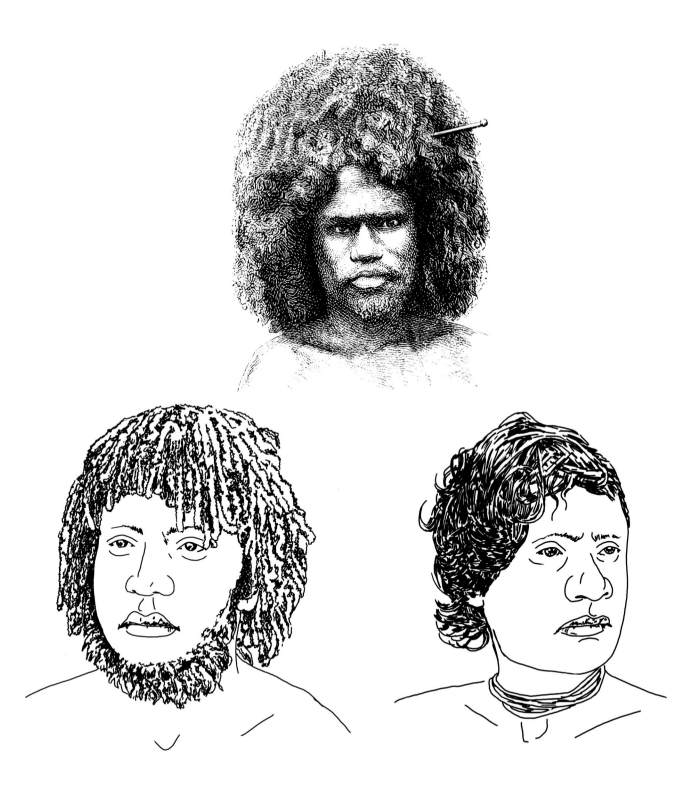

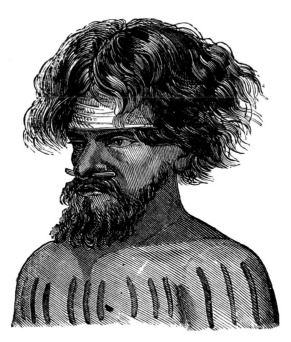

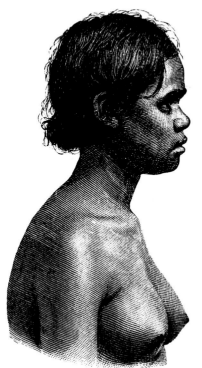

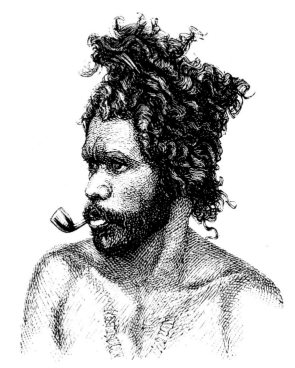

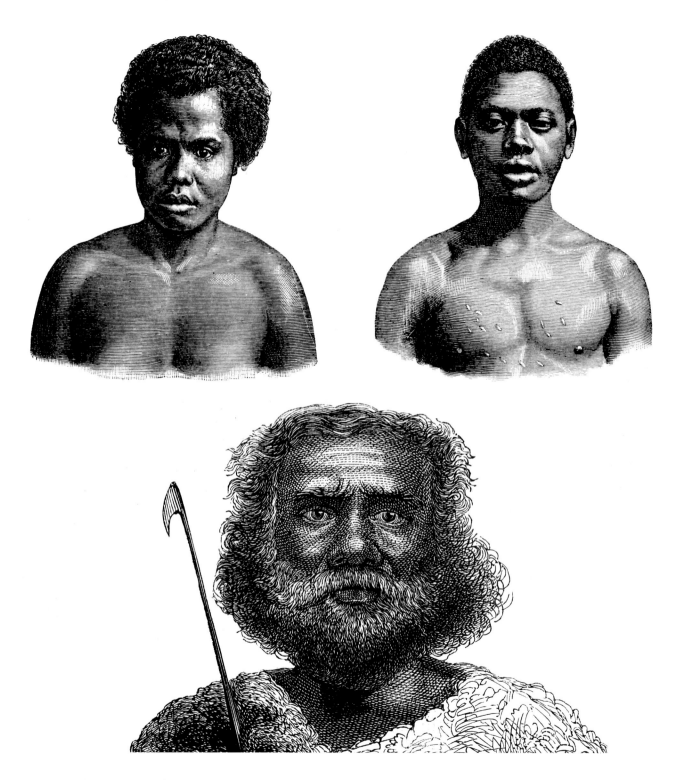

288   Aborigines, Australia

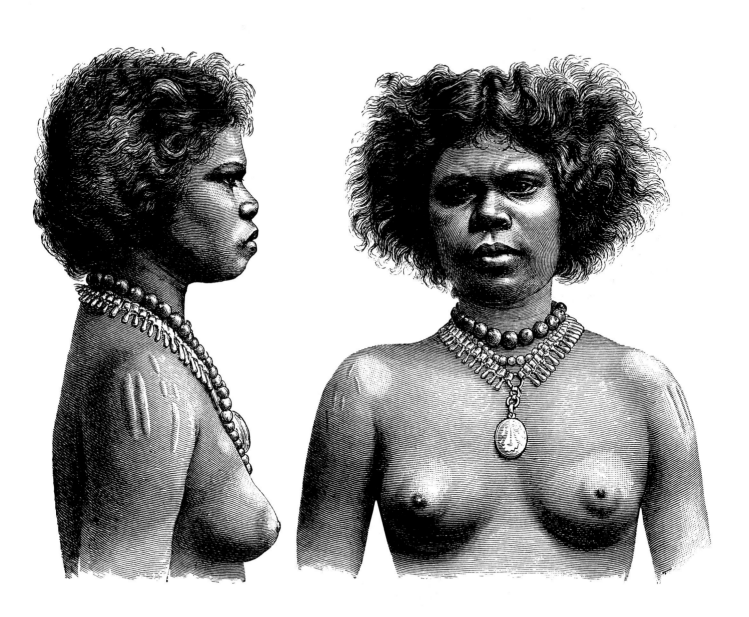

Aborigines, Australia   289

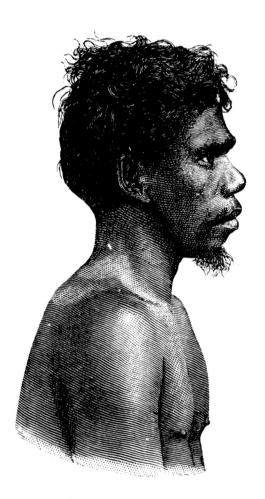
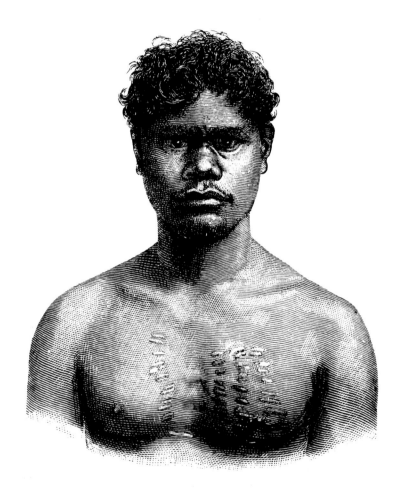

290   Aborigines, Australia

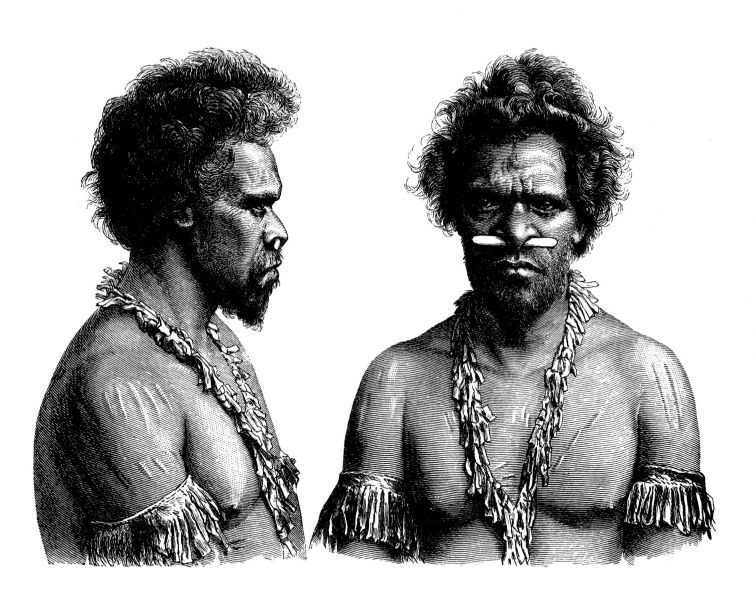

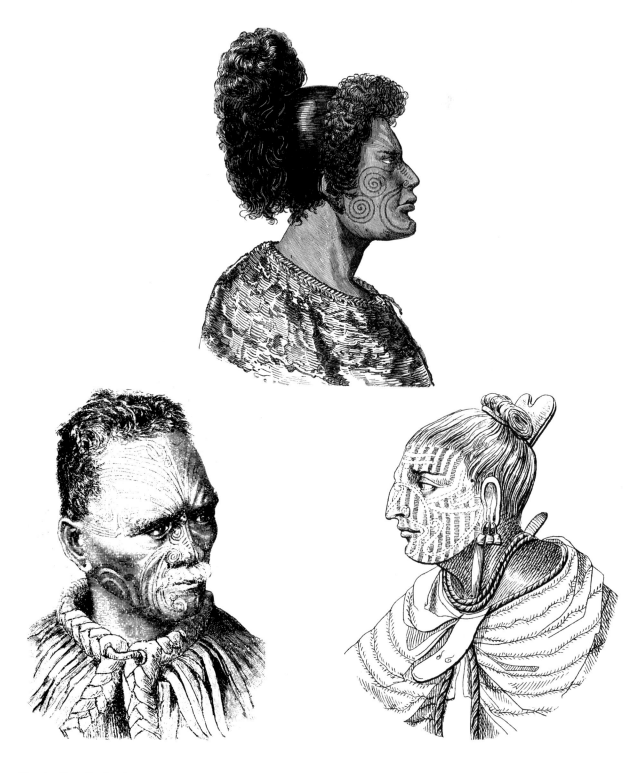

292   Maoris, New Zealand

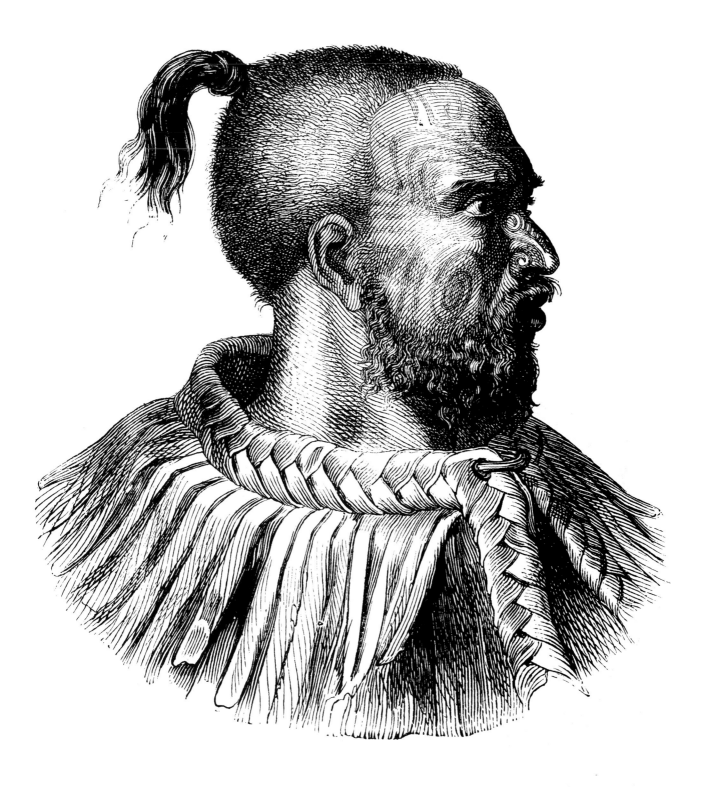

Maori, New Zealand 293

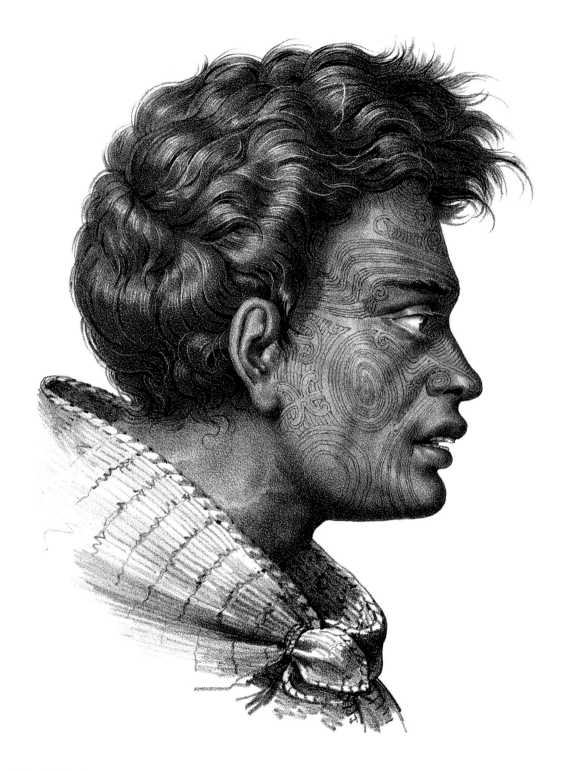

294   Maori, New Zealand

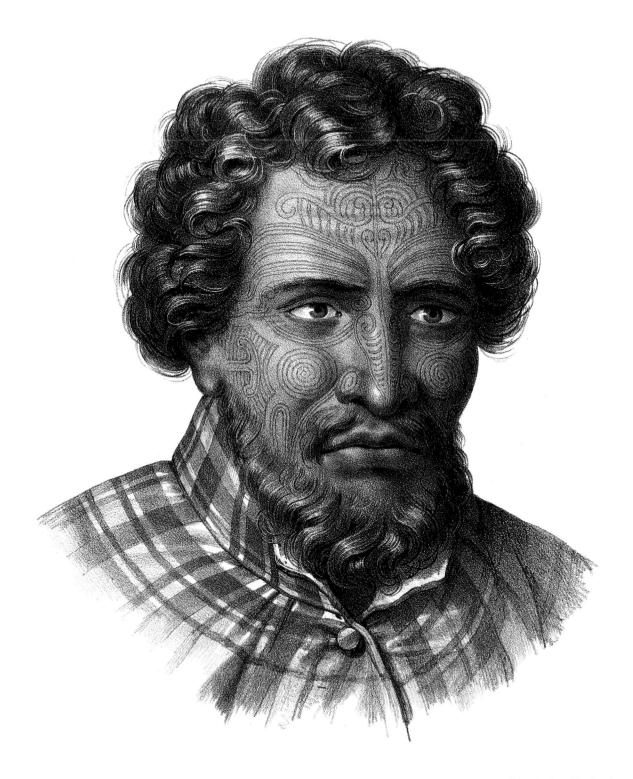

Maori, New Zealand 295

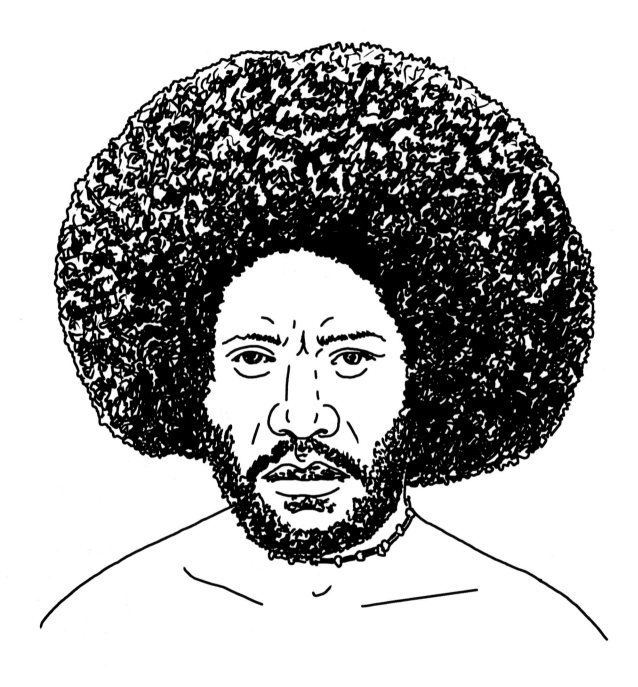

296   Fiji

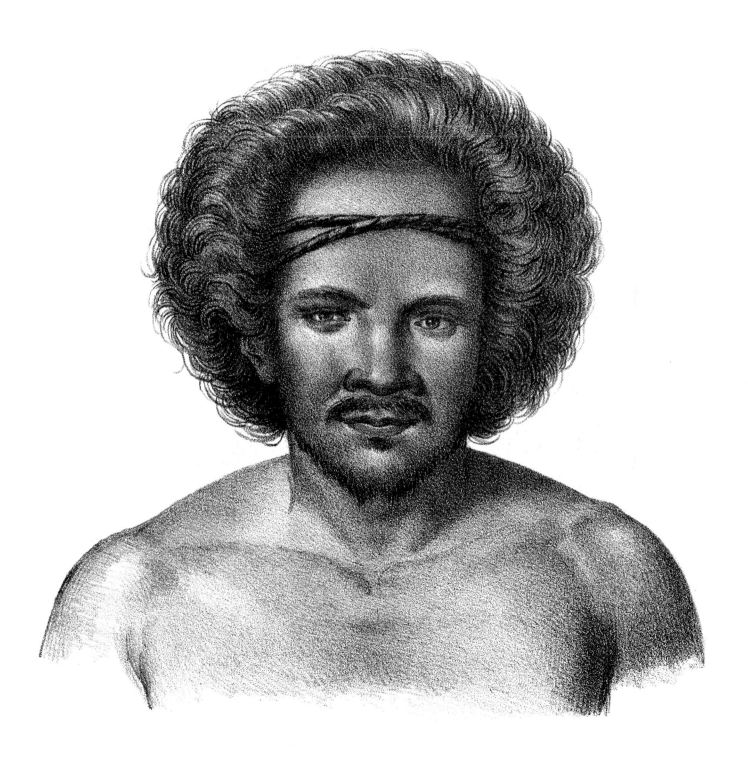

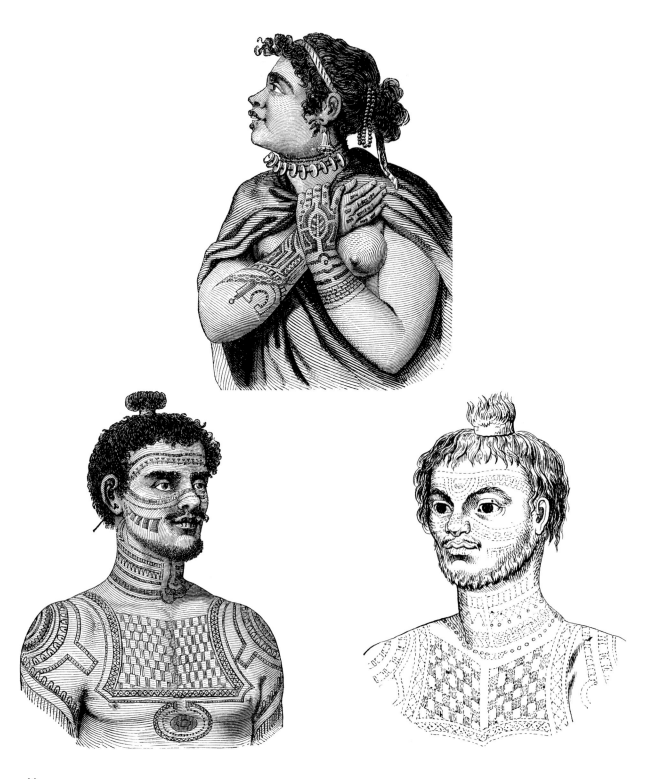

298   Marquesas

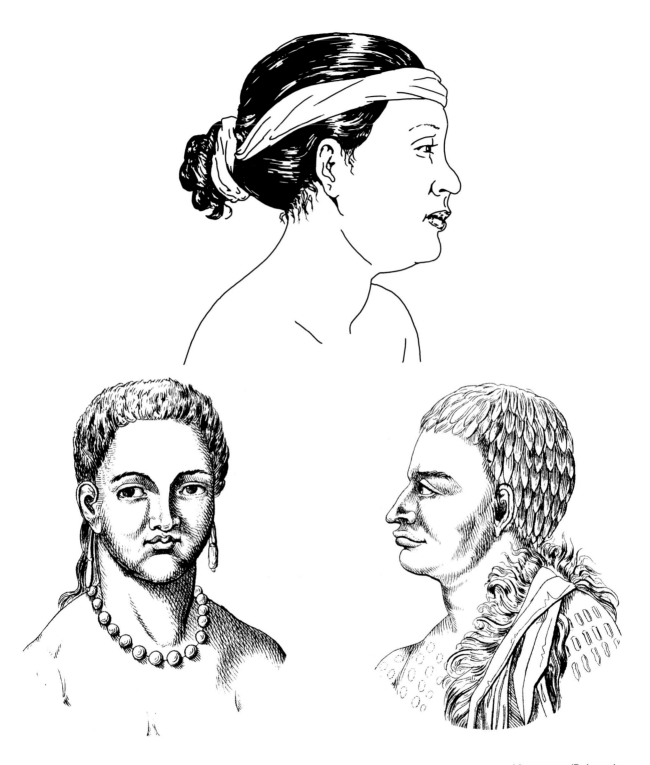

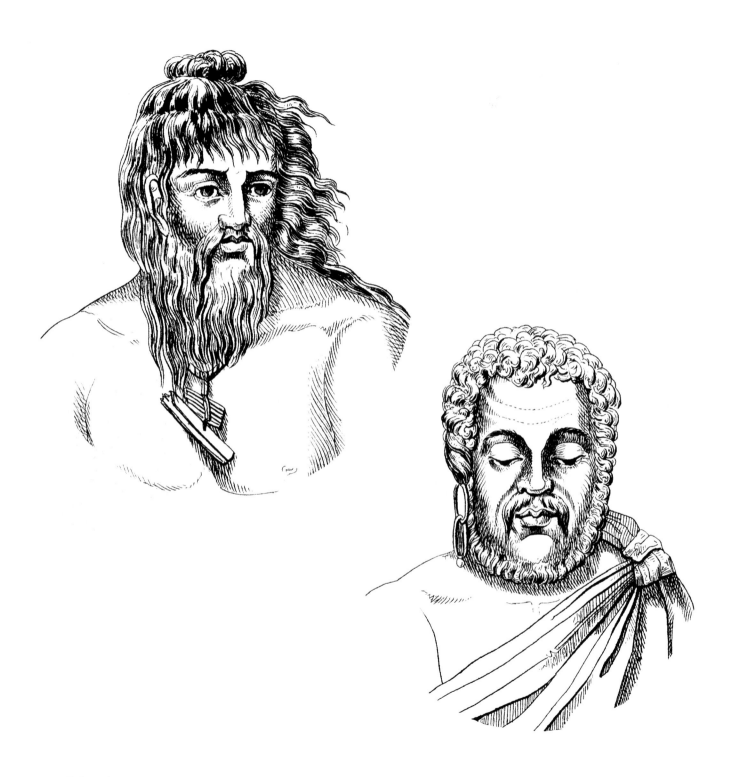

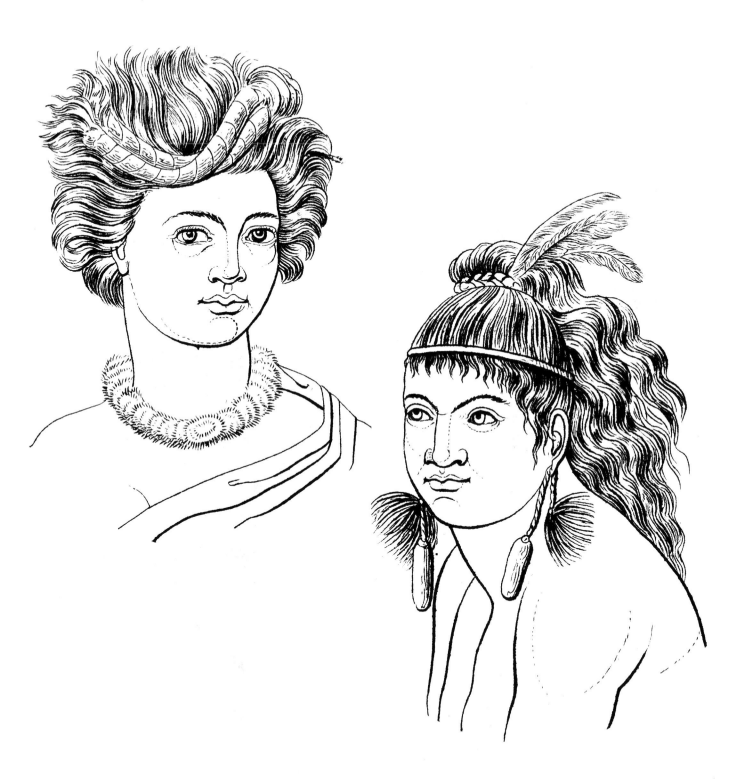

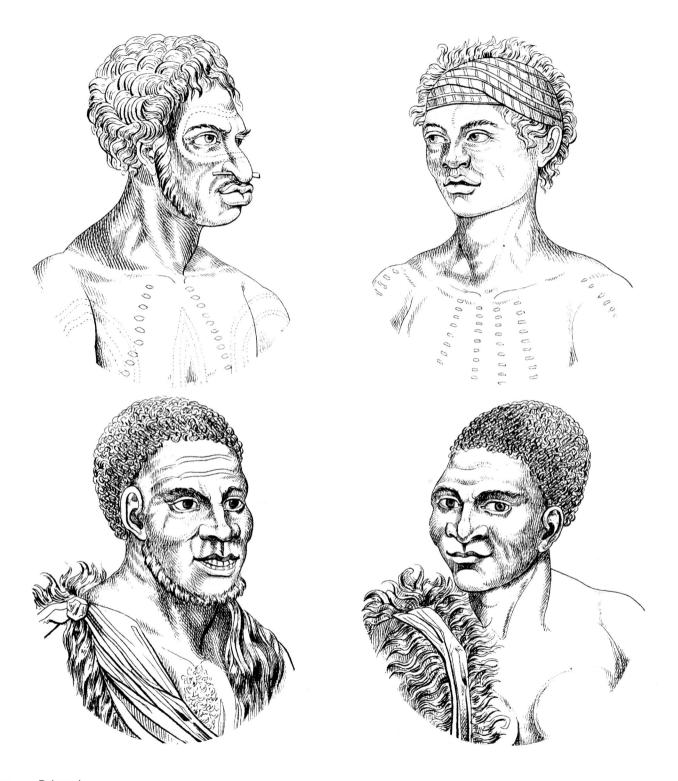

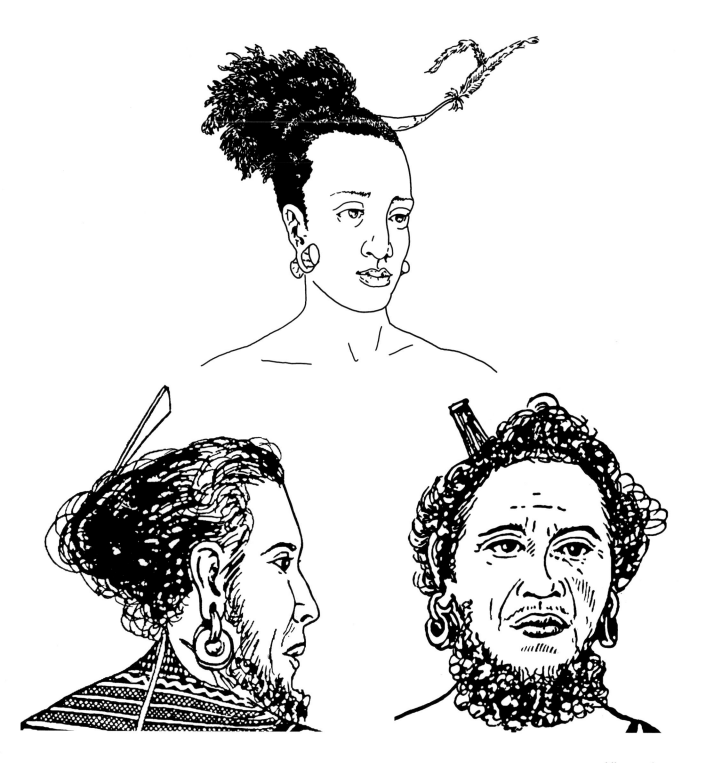

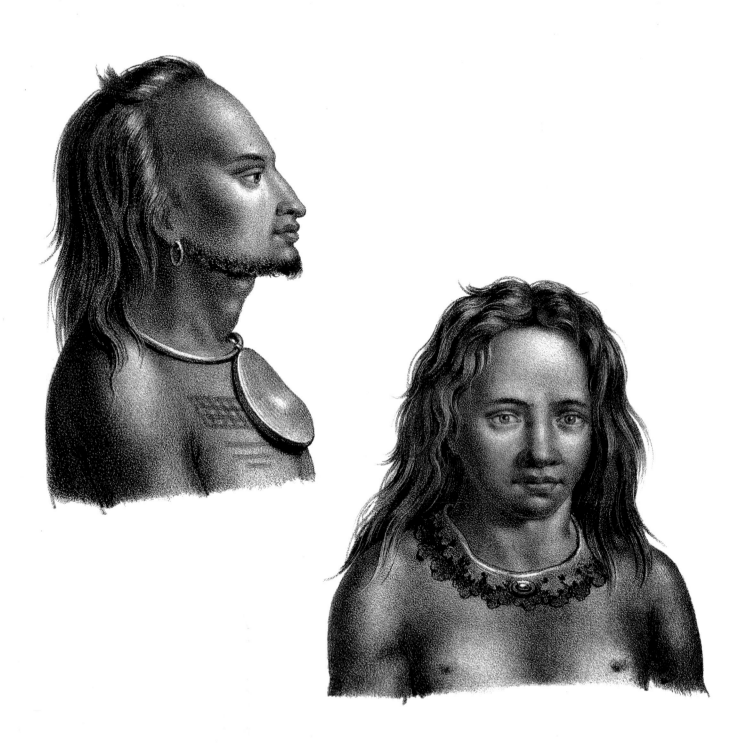

304   Tikopia, Micronesia